DISEASE, KARMA AND HEALING

SPIRITUAL-SCIENTIFIC ENQUIRIES INTO THE
NATURE OF THE HUMAN BEING

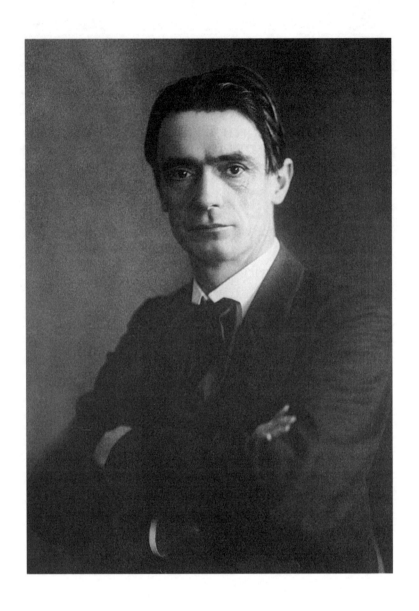

DISEASE, KARMA AND HEALING

SPIRITUAL-SCIENTIFIC ENQUIRIES INTO THE NATURE OF THE HUMAN BEING

Eighteen lectures held in Berlin between October 1908 and June 1909

TRANSLATED BY MATTHEW BARTON

INTRODUCTION BY MATTHEW BARTON

RUDOLF STEINER

RUDOLF STEINER PRESS

CW 107

*The publishers acknowledge the generous funding of this publication by Dr Eva
Frommer MD (1927–2004) and the Anthroposophical Society in
Great Britain*

Rudolf Steiner Press
Hillside House, The Square
Forest Row, RH18 5ES

www.rudolfsteinerpress.com

Published by Rudolf Steiner Press 2013

Originally published in German under the title *Geisteswissenschaftliche Menschenkunde* (volume
107 in the *Rudolf Steiner Gesamtausgabe* or Collected Works) by Rudolf Steiner Verlag,
Dornach. Based on notes taken by members of the audiences not reviewed by the speaker,
and edited by Johann Waeger and Hans W. Zbinden, MD. This authorized translation is
based on the 5th German edition of 2011 which was overseen by David Marc Hoffmann

Published by permission of the Rudolf Steiner Nachlassverwaltung, Dornach

A catalogue record for this book is available from the British Library

ISBN 978 1 85584 383 7

Cover by Mary Giddens
Typeset by DP Photosetting, Neath, West Glamorgan
Printed and bound in Great Britain by Gutenberg Press Ltd., Malta

CONTENTS

Editor's Preface ...... *xiii*

Introduction, by Matthew Barton ...... *xv*

LECTURE 1

BERLIN, 19 OCTOBER 1908

The astral world

The astral world. The streams or currents flowing between human beings and the diverse beings of the astral world. The I as master of the many currents that flow into us. Madness as a consequence of loss of mastery of these currents. Friedrich Nietzsche's madness. The mutual connections between astral beings. Distinctive characteristics of the astral world. Matter's permeability and fruitfulness of ideas as measure of their truth. The two astral worlds, good and bad, and the world of devachan. Kamaloka.

pages 1–13

LECTURE 2

BERLIN, 21 OCTOBER 1908

Some characteristics of the astral world

Repetition as the primary principle of the ether body. Ether body and astral body in plants and animals. Distinctive characteristics of the astral: connection between spatially separated entities (e.g. parallelism in twins), confluence of different astral powers (e.g. Siphonophora), physical development through astral inversion of organs (e.g. organs in fish and humans).

pages 14–26

LECTURE 3

BERLIN, 23 OCTOBER 1908

History of the physical plane and esoteric history

History on the physical plane and esoteric history in the spiritual world. The Atlantean period. The history of decline for the other world and of upsurge for this world. The significance of initiates and of the Mystery of Golgotha in the history of the other world (Christ's descent to hell).

pages 27–38

LECTURE 4

BERLIN, 26 OCTOBER 1908

The law of the astral plane: renunciation. The law of the devachan plane: sacrifice

Objective thinking, feeling and will through esoteric exercises. Feeling, astral vision and Imagination. Will, devachanic hearing (harmony of the spheres) and Inspiration. Privations in the astral world (kamaloca). Renunciation and abstinence as preparation for this. The difference between devachan and the astral world. Bliss in the world of devachan. Sacrifice as preparation for this.

pages 39–47

LECTURE 5

BERLIN, 27 OCTOBER 1908

The nature of pain, suffering, pleasure and bliss

The interplay between etheric and astral. Privation caused by physical injury and suppressed activity of the ether body in the physical body: pain for the astral body. Self-chastisement and asceticism leading to accumulated powers of the etheric body: bliss for the astral body. Savonarola's work as example of the power gained by negating the physical body. Pain in kamaloka, bliss in devachan. Endurance of physical pain as a kind of path of knowledge. The 'crowning with thorns', a stage on the Christian path of initiation as an example of this.

pages 48–53

LECTURE 6

BERLIN, 29 OCTOBER 1908

The four human group souls: lion, bull, eagle and man

Group souls and group egos in Atlantean and Lemurian times. The four group souls of eagle, lion, bull and man and their characters. The gender of the ether body in contrast with that of the physical body. Lion nature and female body, bull nature and male body.

pages 54–61

LECTURE 7

BERLIN, 2 NOVEMBER 1908

Forgetting

Remembering and forgetting. The memory connected with the ether body. The ether body as a principle of repetition. The self-contained lawfulness of the plant ether body. The unused and preserved free part of the human ether body available for education and development. Health and disease and their relationship to the free part of the ether body. The free part of the ether body as precondition for humanity's evolution. How forgotten ideas continually work upon the free part of the ether body. How ideas not forgotten can disrupt development while forgotten ones enhance it. The great blessing of forgetting for daily and ethical/moral life. Learning to forget memories of the physical world in kamaloka (passing through 'Lethe's flood'). The value of forgetting, as indispensable for the good of humanity.

pages 62–72

LECTURE 8

BERLIN, 10 NOVEMBER 1908

The nature of diseases

The inner connections between the lectures in this series. Sickness and healing. Materialistic and spiritual-scientific medicine. The blood as an expression of the I. Five different forms of disease and a few methods of healing: (i) Chronic diseases associated with the blood and the I; the psychological healing method; (ii) acute diseases associated with the nervous system and the astral body; the dietary healing method. (iii) Glandular diseases associated with national characteristics and the ether body; Tabes; the reciprocal relationships between the human organs and between the planets; healing methods using specific medicines (plant, mineral); (iv) infectious diseases associated with the physical body; (v) Diseases associated with human karma; Paracelsus on materialistic physicians.

pages 73–86

LECTURE 9

BERLIN, 16 NOVEMBER 1908

The nature and significance of the Ten Commandments

A translation of the Ten Commandments that takes account of their literal meaning and whole soul import. Yahweh's self-naming as 'I am the I am', and the I of members of the Jewish race. The Yahweh being as a being of transition. The gradual outpouring of knowledge of the I into the Jewish race. The effect of the Ten Commandments on the health of the astral, etheric and physical body. The work of the lower gods to develop the physical, etheric and astral body of the human being, and other nations' veneration of these gods in images. The work of Yahweh on the human I and non-pictorial veneration of him amongst the Jewish people. The few I-aware priests/wise men in other nations, and education of the whole Jewish people, through the Ten Commandments, to be a nation of priests. The I impulse in the Ten Commandments and in the Mystery of Golgotha.

pages 87–101

LECTURE 10
BERLIN, 8 DECEMBER 1908
The nature of original sin

The division of the sexes in Lemurian times and the hermaphrodite beings of the preceding era. People at one with their surroundings in ancient times. Increasing loss of spiritual perceptions. Mutual pleasure of the sexes in each other and the beginning of passionate, sensuous love in the middle of Atlantean times. The Platonic love of former times. Human qualities/characteristics acquired through generations and passed on by inheritance: original sin. Division of the sexes, human individualization and disease. The ungodly nature of the astral body, the more godly nature of the ether body, and the physical body as the temple of God. Mineral medicines and the human phantom (double) they create. The good effects of these medicines: independence of the physical body from harmful influences of the astral and etheric body. The bad effects: weakening of the good influences of the astral and ether body on the physical body.

pages 102–114

LECTURE 11
BERLIN, 21 DECEMBER 1908
The rhythm of the human bodies

The four aspects of the human being during waking and sleeping. Day I and universal I. Rhythmic changes to the I over 24 hours and the relationship between these and the earth's rotation. Astral body and universal astral body. Rhythmic changes to the astral body in seven days, and their relationship to Old Moon and the four lunar phases. Rhythmic changes to the ether body in four times seven days, and their relationship to the lunar orbit. Rhythmic changes to the physical body in ten times seven times four days in the woman, and in twelve times seven times four days in the man, and their relationship to Old Saturn and the earth's orbit. The reciprocal relationships of the four bodies in illness. Fever as exemplified by pneumonia. The rhythms of the four bodies and human freedom. The gradually increasing emancipation from rhythm. Former awareness of these rhythms. Abstraction in materialistic science since the fifteenth century. Medical trials with phenacetin.

pages 115–124

LECTURE 12

BERLIN, 1 JANUARY 1909

Mephistopheles and earthquakes

Mephistopheles and earthquakes. Mephistopheles and Faust's entry into the 'realm of the mothers'. The 'Prologue in Heaven' in *Faust* and the Book of Job in the Old Testament. Who is Mephistopheles? The influence upon us of Lucifer and his associates. Zarathustra and ancient Persian culture. The influence upon us of Ahriman and his associates. Power over fire and earth forces, black magic. Christ's appearance in the other world after the Golgotha event (Christ's descent into hell). Christ fetters Ahriman. The Asuras. Ongoing connection of the whole karma of humanity with the karma of Ahriman. Individual karma and the karma of all humanity. The layers of the earth. The sixth layer (fire earth) as the centre of Ahriman's activity. Earthquakes and volcanic eruptions as reverberations of the Lemurian and Atlantean catastrophes. The possibility, difficulties of and justification for esoterically predicting earthquakes.

pages 125–143

LECTURE 13

BERLIN, 12 JANUARY 1909

Rhythms in human nature

The rhythms of I, astral body, ether body and physical body in the ratio of $1:7:(4 \times 7):(10 \times 4 \times 7)$. Fever as the organism's defence against illness. The lungs. The mutual relationship between diverse rhythms of ether body and astral body. The movements of heavenly bodies and of the rhythms of the human bodies. The rhythm of the physical body (10×28 days $= 10$ sidereal months) and the period between human conception and birth. The thinking of the angels in harmony with the rhythms of the cosmos; the arrhythmic nature of human thinking and feeling.

Human independence from the ancient, external rhythm, and the development of a new, inner rhythm. Reciprocal relationship of the human bodies, and of the earth's incarnations, in a 4:7 ratio.

pages 144–157

LECTURE 14

BERLIN, 26 JANUARY 1909

Disease and karma

Disease and death. The period in kamaloca. Hindrances and obstacles in life as a possibility for self-overcoming and strengthening. Redress in subsequent lives for pain and harm we have caused in former times. Inadequacy of inherited forces (incarnation) in relation to karmic powers and requirements of the soul as a reason for disharmony in human nature. The karmic causes of diseases. Disease and recovery as strengthening and preparation for karmic redress that is not yet possible but will later be realized. Health and illness before and during Lemurian times. The rites of Asclepius in Greek mythology.

pages 158–171

LECTURE 15

BERLIN, 15 FEBRUARY 1909

Christianity in the evolution of modern humanity. Leading individualities and avatars

The evolution of the human being through diverse incarnations, in contrast to the evolution of avatars. Christ as the greatest avatar. The workings of avatars on earth. The connection between an avatar and the ether body of Shem, the progenitor of the Semites. The countless multiplied images of this ether body in Shem's physical descendants. The preservation of Shem's own ether body in the world of spirit for Melchizedek's special task in relation to the Hebrew people's mission. Melchizedek's impulse in relation to Abraham. The multiplication of the ether body, astral body and I of Jesus of Nazareth through the entry of the Christ avatar into Jesus. The preservation of these multiplied ether and astral bodies in the spiritual world and their later interweaving into human beings mature enough for this. The intimate history of Christian development relating to this: first to fifth centuries; the great value of physical memories of the working of Christ and the Apostles. Examples: Irenaeus, Papias, Augustine of Hippo. Fourth to twelfth centuries: clairvoyant revelations of the events in Palestine through the multiplied ether bodies of Jesus of Nazareth interwoven into many people. Example: the author of the Heliand poem. Eleventh to fifteenth centuries: religious fervour and direct conviction through the [multiplied] astral bodies of Jesus of Nazareth interwoven into the most important proponents of Christianity. Examples for the sentient soul: Francis of Assisi, Franciscans, Elisabeth of Thuringia; for the mind soul: scholastics; for the consciousness soul: mystics Johannes Tauler, Meister Eckhart. Fifteenth to sixteenth centuries: development of modern science from medieval Christian science. Sixteenth to twentieth centuries: preparation of the I to become a Christ-receptive organ through spiritual science.

pages 172–187

LECTURE 16

BERLIN, 22 MARCH 1909

The deed of Christ and the adversary powers of Lucifer, Ahriman and the Asuras

The spirits that help human evolution to progress, and the adversarial, inhibiting spiritual beings. The influence of luciferic beings in Lemurian times: sensory desire. The remedy of the progressive spirits: illness, suffering, pain and death. The influence of the ahrimanic spirits in Atlantean times: error and sin. The remedy: the powers of karma as the possibility of correcting error and sin. The influence of Lucifer and Ahriman today: Lucifer in the sentient soul, Ahriman in the mind soul. The forthcoming, much more intense power of evil of the Asuras in the consciousness soul and the I. The difficulty of expiating the evil of the Asuras. Christ as giver of the possibility of karma. The loss of direct vision of the spiritual world due to the influence of Lucifer and Ahriman. The redemption of luciferic beings by human Christ perception. The resurrected, purified and cleansed luciferic spirit as Holy Spirit. The meaning of the Holy Spirit in the lodge of the Masters of Wisdom and of the Harmony of Feelings, and in human Christ perception. The real, positive power of spiritual science. The supposed opposition between eastern and western esotericism.

pages 188–204

LECTURE 17

BERLIN, 27 APRIL 1909

Laughing and weeping. The physiognomy of the divine in human beings

Laughing and weeping in the human being, compared with grinning and howling in the animal. Weeping as the expression of a certain disharmony with the outer world, as compression of the astral body by the I. Laughing as expanding of the astral body by the I. Individual nature of the human being, group soul and group I in the animal. The reversal of breathing processes in laughing and weeping. Laughing and weeping as expression of human egohood. Laughing as a sense of superiority over something. Weeping as cowering and withdrawing into oneself. Unnecessary and unjustified laughing and weeping. The right balance between joy and pain: caused neither by arrogance nor by being compressed but by the relationship between I and environment. Smiling through tears, weeping through laughter. Laughter and tears as expression of the physiognomy of the divine in human beings.

pages 205–217

LECTURE 18
BERLIN, 17 JUNE 1909
Evolution, involution and creation out of nothing

Human evolution as distinct from the evolution of animal and plant. The death of the plant following sexual maturation after developing and unfolding its ether body. The death of the animal following development and unfolding of the astral body. The developmental capacity of the human I from incarnation to incarnation, and in relation to education. An example of developmental realities: the seed and the full-grown flower, involution and evolution. Evolution and involution in the human being between birth and death, and between death and birth. The difference compared with the plant: the possibility of creating out of nothing, of experiences not determined by karma. Creating the human being anew for Venus evolution through creating out of nothing. The human I elevates itself: (i) through logical thinking; (ii) through aesthetic judgement; (iii) through moral judgement and fulfilment of duties. The participation of the Spirits of Personality (Time Spirits) in this human evolution. The creation of the true, the beautiful and the good out of nothing as creation in the Holy Spirit. The entry of Christ into our evolution as foundation for this. The incarnation of Christ in a human body as a free deed, as creation out of nothing.

pages 218–236

Notes 237

Rudolf Steiner's Collected Works 242

Significant Events in the Life of Rudolf Steiner 256

Index 271

EDITOR'S PREFACE

'This cycle of lectures over the past winter has dealt with anthropology in the broadest sense, with a study of humankind, and this subject will be one that continues to preoccupy us in the most varied fields.'

Rudolf Steiner, 3 May 1909

After the German section of the Theosophical Society was founded in October 1902 with Rudolf Steiner as its general secretary, the latter began to give a series of 'ongoing lectures covering the whole field of theosophy' as a continually deepening introduction to theosophy for members of the Berlin branch—at that time also known as a 'lodge'. The 18 members' lectures comprising this volume, given during the so-called 'winter semester' of 1908/1909, follow on organically from lecture series for the Berlin branch (dissolved in 1906) and the 'Besant branch' which Rudolf Steiner and Marie Steiner founded in 1905.

Since Rudolf Steiner could assume that his audience was familiar with the works he had so far published—*Theosophy, Knowledge of the Higher Worlds* and *The Stages of Higher Knowledge* — this now gave him a basis for developing more differentiated esoteric studies of the human being, the earth and the cosmos. The title of the original German edition of this volume—'Spiritual-Scientific Enquiries into the Nature of the Human Being'—was very probably chosen for this series of lectures with Rudolf Steiner's endorsement, and is very apposite for their unifying theme.

Two further aspects to which Rudolf Steiner drew attention are also important for understanding these lectures. He reminds his audience of the public lectures he was giving during the same period at the Architects' House, *Wo und wie findet man den Geist?* (GA 57, 'Where and How Do We Find the Spirit?', not translated): 'We can only ascend to ever higher domains in these meetings here by arranging the courses running parallel to these branch lectures in the way that we have. I would therefore ask you to take note of these courses as far as you can.' For readers today, likewise, it is very illuminating to study these two lecture series alongside each other, and to note the difference in mode of presentation between those for a public audience and those for members. At the same time it was very important to Rudolf Steiner that previously published lecture transcripts should be read—if at all—in the sequence in which they were given, since he had placed them in an intrinsically coherent sequence (see also the lecture of 10 November 1908, page 102).

INTRODUCTION

Today illness is almost universally regarded as a nuisance at best, and at worst a grave misfortune. It is not therefore largely seen as intrinsic to our human state but as a troubling anomaly, a deviation from the norm of health, which must if possible be fiercely combated. Modern medicine seeks to do this with all the weapons and knowledge in its armoury. No one could possibly argue with the medical profession's ethical, laudable efforts to provide remedies and alleviate suffering. But, as becomes clear in many places in this volume, illness and suffering can also be seen in a much larger context. Steiner states that 'What has been gained from one angle needs enlarging and extending through insight from another' (lecture 4). While he is referring here to his own efforts to approach reality from many diverse, complementary perspectives, this statement can also readily apply to the way we normally view disease. Our view of it can be enlarged and extended by understanding—as Steiner seeks to show— that disease and illness also offer us a 'path of knowledge', confronting us with hindrances, weaknesses and obstacles that we need to engage with to progress. This very word 'progress' at the same time begs further questions of our development as human beings, both in this life on earth and beyond death into future stages of our evolution. While 'suffering' an illness we may of course die. But, according to Steiner, it will still have given us the strength to realize and more fully embody our karma in a subsequent life. In this view, illness is a misfortune only from a narrower and more immediate perspective. From a larger, complementary one, it offers us the opportunity for deeper healing. It is itself a 'remedy' to balance our otherwise deep immersion in sensory delights of the material world, reminding us, also, of the pain and curtailments of merely physical existence. William Blake famously wrote:

Joy and woe are woven fine,
A clothing for the soul divine,
Under every grief and pine,
Runs a joy with silken twine.

It is right it should be so,
We were made for joy and woe,
And when this we rightly know,
Through the world we safely go.

Joy and pain both belong to our lives as embodied spiritual beings. And illness can be a *salutary* reminder in the truest sense, without which we might so easily lose sight of the distinctive nature of our humanity, which is our conscious connection with worlds of spirit. Today's prevailing paradigm of materialism is at present mostly only a belief, though one very strongly held in many quarters. While many think, for instance, that 'our loftiest ethical ideas are just highly developed animal drives' (lecture 16), they do not on the whole live according to this belief but still hold to a sense of their humanity and their capacity to act in free and moral ways. We do however gradually create our own reality, and Steiner warns that the materialistic outlook urgently needs enlarging with insight into the workings of spirit within matter; with, for instance, the idea and experience of karma and of the non-material realities that inform our physical lives. Problems come to expression in the physical body but mostly do not originate in it. In Steiner's own metaphor, considering the physical body alone in efforts to cure illness is rather like tinkering with a train engine when the problem actually lies with the train driver. Part of a physician's work, in fact, involves gaining insight into the whole nature of an individual, his core being. Ultimately, says Steiner, the health of individual human beings and of humanity as a whole will depend on a redemptive knowledge of the whole compass of our nature, including spiritual aspects that—like the larger part of the iceberg hidden beneath the surface—are no less real for being, at present, hard to discern.

Hard but not impossible. Throughout this volume Steiner seeks to draw our attention to the greater scope of the smallest phenomena— even a seemingly insignificant headache for instance. He casts vivid light on things we usually take for granted, such as the human capacity—not shared with animals—to laugh or cry; and in the process he enormously broadens our vision of human existence. Similarly he shows how the apparently mundane human experiences of forgetting and remembering are intrinsic to our humanity and have unsuspected moral and spiritual dimensions. Thus Steiner's insights are never merely 'lofty' or nebulously 'spiritual' but time and again connect with the minutest realities of everyday life and the particularities of the human condition. He himself demonstrates what he continually urges upon us: that the spirit is everywhere the *primum mobile* giving rise to all phenomena in the world. At the same time it becomes clear that we are distinguished from the animal kingdom by the core identity of the 'I' we bear within us, which embodies our capacity to learn, change and progress by our own intrinsic, developing powers so that we can become free, and freely creative, in ways that animals are not. This, for Steiner, is the very essence of the two necessarily connected phenomena of human health and illness: a view in which physical and spiritual health become identical, and cannot be sundered from a far-reaching vista of human evolution. Ultimately we are not just the product of this evolution, of the blind working of natural forces, but can gradually become the free creators of our own nature and destiny.

Matthew Barton, September 2013

LECTURE 1

W E have gathered here for several previous winter courses to consider spiritual-scientific themes. A few of you have already taken part in quite a number of these winter gatherings of ours. For reasons we will perhaps come to speak of during the forthcoming annual general meeting,[1] this moment is an apt one for casting our minds back a little to the anthroposophical endeavours we have so far engaged in together. In a sense, several of you still form a kind of core of this gathering and have brought your fundamental spiritual conviction with you from earlier studies. Six or seven years ago you joined us to form the core around which, if one can put it like this, all our other questing friends have gradually crystallized.[2] And it is telling that these gatherings have not only grown in numerical terms over this period but that, with the aid of the spiritual powers always present when spiritual-scientific work is accomplished in the right way, we have also succeeded in remaining inwardly systematic in our work to some degree.

Those especially who have taken part in our branch meetings from the very beginning may reflect on how we started as a small group six or seven years ago, and how very slowly and gradually, and also inwardly, in terms of inner content we have created the ground upon which we stand today. We started with the simplest spiritual-scientific concepts, trying to create a foundation for ourselves; and gradually we arrived at the point when, last winter—at least in our branch meetings—it became possible to speak of various aspects of the higher worlds in the same way as one speaks of events and experiences in the mundane physical world. We were able to learn about diverse spiritual entities and the worlds which are supersensible by contrast to our sensory world. Besides cultivating an inwardly consistent and systematic approach in our branch work, it also proved possible to give two courses last winter[3] during which those who had gradually assembled around the core group could as it were pick up the thread of our ongoing studies.

Those of our members who can recall the beginnings of our present branch group will also remember various difficulties and obstacles in this work. Throughout all such difficulties, some among you kept faith with what we call spiritual-scientific work. Those who know how to endure faithfully, patiently and energetically will, sooner or later, come to see that faithfulness and energy bring certain results.

As mentioned, and often emphasized here, we have ultimately succeeded in speaking of higher worlds as something self-evident, and have stressed that those who inwardly participated in our branch gatherings over a longer period have acquired a certain anthroposophical maturity in consequence. Such maturity does not lie in a theoretical domain, in some kind of conceptual understanding, but rather in an inner mood one can acquire over time. Anyone who for a while really inwardly absorbs what spiritual science can offer will gradually come to feel that he can listen to things as realities, real facts, as something self-evident, which he would previously have experienced in a quite different way.

Today, then, in this introductory lecture, let us immediately start to speak in an unconstrained and even uninhibited way of a certain aspect of the higher worlds which can bring us to deeper understanding of human character and personality. Basically, what is served by all the considerations we give here to higher worlds? When we speak about the astral world, or the world of devachan, in what sense, as inhabitants of the physical world, are we initially speaking? In speaking of these higher worlds, we have no sense whatever that they are something wholly alien to us, and have no connection with the physical world. No, we are aware that what we refer to as 'higher worlds' surround us, that we live within them, that these higher worlds permeate our physical world and that these higher worlds contain the active causes and originating foundations of realities which unfold here before our physical eyes and physical senses. Thus we only come to know the life which surrounds us, in its relationship to us and natural phenomena, if we regard this invisible life—manifesting, though, in the visible realm—as part of other worlds, and can therefore assess how it plays into our physical world. Both normal and abnormal phenomena of ordinary physical life only become clear to us when we familiarize ourselves with the spiritual life underlying the physical—this spiritual life far richer and more encompassing than physical life, which represents only a small part of it.

The human being is the focus of all our considerations—and must be so. To understand the human being really means understanding a great part of the world itself. But it is hard to understand him. However, we will acquire a little insight into the human being if we speak today of just a few—among the enormous number—of facts relating to what we call the astral world. As you know, the content of the human soul is very rich and diverse. Today let us bring to mind a portion of this soul content: let us consider certain qualities of soul.

In our soul life we live within the fullest range of feelings and emotions, and in thoughts, images, ideas and will impulses. From morning to evening all this unfolds in our life of soul. If we observe the human being in a superficial way, this soul life rightly appears to us as self-contained, as inwardly consistent. Just consider how your life flows by: how in the morning you entertain the first thought of the day, and the first emotion flickers through your soul, your first will impulse emerges. And consider how, until consciousness sinks into sleep again at night, idea after idea, feeling after feeling, will impulse after will impulse continually succeed one another. All this appears like a steady flow. From a deeper perspective, though, this is not such a continuous flow for we are always connected with higher worlds—though most people are unaware of this—through our thoughts, feelings and sentience. Today let us consider this relationship of ours with the astral world.

When we have some feeling or other, when joy or alarm flare in our soul, initially this is an occurrence within our soul. But it is not merely that. If one is able to examine this clairvoyantly, it becomes apparent that something like a luminous stream emanates from a person at the moment of alarm or joy, and that this enters the astral world. It does not enter it haphazardly or arbitrarily, though, but makes its way to a being within the astral world. In other words, when a feeling shimmers up in us, we enter into a connection with a being of the astral world. Let us assume that some thought occupies a place in our soul. Let's say that we reflect on the nature of a table. As this thought quivers through our soul, the clairvoyant can demonstrate how a current issues from this thought and seeks out a being of the astral world. And the same is true of every thought, every mental picture, every emotion. From the whole current of life that issues from the soul, streams continually flow towards the most diverse beings of the astral world. It would be quite wrong to think that these outflowing streams all went to a *single* being in the astral world. This is not so. Instead, the most varied currents stream from all these separate thoughts, emotions and feelings, and connect with the most diverse beings of the astral world. This is the remarkable thing here: that as individuals we are not connected with just a *single* such being, but that we spin the most diverse threads connecting us to the most diverse beings of the astral world. The astral world is populated by a large number of entities just as the physical world is; and these beings are connected with us in the most varied and diverse ways.

But if we wish to gain insight into the full complexity of this, we also have to consider something else. Let us assume that two people see a flash of lightning and both have a very similar feeling in response to it. From each of the two a current emanates, but both these now flow to one and the same being in the astral world. We can say therefore that there is a being, an inhabitant of the astral world, with whom the two beings of the physical world establish a connection. It may be that not just one but 50, 100 or 1000 human beings have similar sentiments or perceptions and emit currents which stream towards a single being of the astral world. In uniting in this one point, these thousand human beings establish a connection with the same being of the astral world. But now picture the other different emotions, feelings and thoughts which these people—who share the same emotion in this one instance— carry within them! Through these other currents they are connected with other entities in the astral world, and in consequence the most diverse connecting threads pass from the astral world into the physical world.

Now it is possible to distinguish certain categories of beings in the astral world. We gain an idea of these different classes most easily if we consider the following example. Take a large number of Europeans and examine for a moment the concept or idea of justice contained in their souls. People may otherwise have the most varied experiences and therefore connect with the most diverse beings of the astral world in the most intricate and complex ways. But when these people think about the concept of justice in the same way, appropriate it in the same way, they all connect with one being of the astral world; and we can regard this being of the astral world really as a centre, a focal point, from which issue rays towards all those who share this idea. Whenever such people call to mind their concept of justice, they are connected with this single being. Just as we have flesh and blood, and are composed of it, so this being is constituted of the concept of justice: it lives within it. Likewise there are astral beings for the concepts of courage, benevolence, fortitude, revenge and so forth. So you see that qualities we can have as human beings, the contents of our soul, correspond to beings in the astral world. This means that something like an astral net spreads out over a larger number of people. All of us who share the same concepts of justice are embedded in the body of an astral entity whom we could really call the being of justice. All of us who share the same concepts of courage, fortitude and so forth, are connected with one and the same astral being, constituted of, and embodying, justice, courage or fortitude. Thus each one of us is a kind of conglomeration of streams—for we can regard each person as receiving from all directions streams sent out by astral beings. All of us are a confluence of streams entering us from the astral world.

During the winter lectures we will increasingly be able to show how the human being is basically a confluence of streams as I have described, and focuses these streams within him, around the central point of his I. You see, the most important thing for human soul life is that we concentrate all these streams around a focal point which lies within our self-awareness. This self-awareness is so important in us since it must hold sway like a ruler in our inner human entelechy, encompassing and connecting the diverse streams that flow into us from all sides. Were self-awareness to lapse, the human being might immediately cease to feel himself a unity, and all the diverse concepts of courage, fortitude and so forth might then fall asunder. A person would then cease to have the sense of being a unity but would instead feel himself sundered into all the different streams. A person can in a sense lose directing mastery over what streams into him—and here we see how we can gain understanding of the spiritual world through insight into the real state of affairs. Consider that as a single individual you have lived a particular kind of life, experiencing various things, and from youth onwards nurturing a number of ideals which gradually developed in you. Every such ideal can be different from another. You have had the ideal of courage, fortitude, benevolence and so forth, thereby entering into streams from the most diverse astral beings. There is also another way in which we can engage with a diverse succession of streams from astral beings. Assume we have had a number of friendships during our life. Very particular feelings and emotions will have developed under the influence of these friendships, especially during our youth. In this way, streams went out to a quite specific being in the astral world. Then a new friendship entered our life, connecting us therefore with a different being of the astral world—and so on, throughout life. Now let us assume that the psyche suffered disturbance so that the I lost mastery over the various different streams and was no longer able to hold them together. We would arrive at a state when we ceased to feel ourselves as an I, as an intact entity, as a unity within our self-awareness. If we were to lose our I through a process of mental illness, we would no longer experience these streams as something through which we perceive ourselves but as if we were flowing out and dissolving into them. Certain cases of mental illness only become comprehensible when we consider them from this perspective, that of the astral world. One such case is Friedrich Nietzsche.[4]

Many of you will probably have heard that Friedrich Nietzsche suffered an outbreak of madness during the winter of 1888/1889. Readers of his last letters will find it interesting to observe how Friedrich Nietzsche fragmented into diverse streams at the moment when he lost his I. For instance, he writes to this or that friend, or also notes to himself: 'A god lives in Turin who was once a professor of philosophy in Basel, but he was not egotistical enough to remain so.'[5] In other words, he had lost his I, and he clothed this fact in words such as these. 'And the god Dionysus walks by the Po.'[6] And he looks down on all his ideals and friendships, which wander below him. Sometimes he thinks he is King Carlo Alberto,[7] at other times someone else, sometimes even one of the criminals he was reading about during the last days of his life. At this time there were two murder cases which had attracted much attention, and at moments in his illness he identified with those lady-killers. He no longer experienced his I but instead a stream flowing into the astral world. In abnormal cases, therefore, separate currents otherwise made to cohere by our centre of self-awareness rise to the surface of life.

It will become ever more necessary for people to know what lies in the depths of the soul. You see, we would be endlessly impoverished if we were unable to produce many such streams that enter the astral world; and our nature would be very restricted if we were unable, by deepening our lives spiritually, to gain mastery over all these streams. We really must say therefore that we are not confined within our skin but extend beyond it on all sides into other worlds, which in turn penetrate into our world. A whole network of entities is spun out over the astral world.

Now let us examine in a little more detail a few of these entities that are connected with us in this way. These are beings that present themselves to us roughly as follows. The astral world surrounds us. Let us conceive of such a being, say the one relating to the concept and feeling of courage. It stretches its tentacles out in all directions, and these tentacles enter human souls. As people develop courage a connection is created between this being of courage and the human soul. Other people are different. All, for instance, who develop a certain kind of feeling of love or anxiety are connected with a being of the astral world. When we engage with these beings we enter into what we can say constitutes life in the astral world, its social coherence. As people live here on the physical plane they are not merely separate beings. Here on the physical plane, too, we are involved in hundredfold and thousandfold interconnections. We have legal arrangements with one another, and are involved in friendships and suchlike. Our connections on the physical plane are governed by our ideas, concepts, mental pictures and so on. In a certain sense, the social connections of the beings we have been considering on the astral plane must likewise be governed in some way. So how do these beings coexist with each other? They do not have a dense, physical body of flesh and blood as we do; instead they have astral bodies, are composed at most of etheric substance. They stretch out their feelers into our world. But how do they live together? If these beings did not collaborate, our human life would also be quite different. Basically, our physical world is only the external expression of what occurs on the astral plane. Picture a being in the astral world, the being of justice, to whom stream all thoughts relating to justice; then picture another, to whom flow all thoughts relating to giving. If the idea forms in our soul that giving is justice, then a stream issues from both these beings and enters our soul. We are connected with both. But how do these two beings bear with one another?

One might be tempted to think that social or communal coexistence on the astral plane is the same as on the physical plane, yet it is different in very important respects. It is wrong merely to place the different planes one above the other and characterize what happens in the higher worlds as closely resembling occurrences in the physical world. There is a huge difference between the physical world and the higher worlds, one which becomes ever greater the higher we ascend. Above all, the astral world is distinguished by a singular quality that cannot be found on the physical plane at all. This is the permeability, the penetrability of the matter of the astral plane. In the physical world it is impossible for you to stand at exactly the same place as another person—and thus impenetrability is a law of the physical world. This is not true in the astral world, and there the law of permeability prevails. There it is certainly possible, and even the usual thing, for beings to interpenetrate, for one being to enter the space already occupied by another. Two, four, a hundred beings can be at one and the same place simultaneously in the astral world. What this means though, in turn, is that the logic of communal coexistence is quite different on the astral plane from the physical plane. You can best grasp the nature of this different logic—not the logic of thinking but that of action—if you consider the following example.

Imagine that a city council decided to build a church at a certain location. The council would inevitably first have to discuss how to build it, how to organize this and so on. Now let's assume there are two groups on the council, and that the two have different ideas about architecture and the choice of building company. On the physical plane the two parties will be at loggerheads and unable to carry out their plans until one of them gets the upper hand and carries the day, securing agreement as to the design of the church. You are aware of course that the great majority of human social interactions involve such discussion and negotiation before anything is realized, so that people can first agree about what should actually be done. Nothing at all would get done unless, in most cases, one party prevailed and secured a majority. The minority party will not easily concede that it was in the wrong, but instead will go on believing it was right. In the physical world, we are involved therefore in discussion about ideas that must be decided purely within this physical world, since it is impossible for two different plans to be realized at one and the same location.

In the astral world things are completely different. There it would be perfectly possible to build, say, two churches at one and the same place. In fact such things continually occur in the astral world, and this alone is the right and proper thing there. Disputes do not occur there as they do in the physical world. Meetings are not held where a majority opinion is sought for this or that venture, nor is there any need at all for this. When a council meeting takes place and 40 out of 45 councillors have one view while the others have another, it is not so dire if the two parties feel like murdering each other because of their differences of opinion, since these things come to immediate outward expression, are voiced. One party will not try to build its church without regard to the other, since on the physical plane a thought can remain a content of the soul: it can remain within us. Things are not so straightforward on the astral plane. There, when an idea is formed, in a certain sense it *already exists*. Thus if an astral being such as those I have been speaking of has a thought, it immediately extends the corresponding feelers which have the form of this thought, while another extends its own feelers; and both interpenetrate and now exist in the same space as a newly formed entity.

Thus the most diverse opinions, thoughts and feelings continually interpenetrate. The most contrary things can interpenetrate in the astral world. While disagreement occurs in the physical world about such things as we have mentioned, in the astral world actual conflict immediately arises. You see, as beings in the astral world you cannot restrain a thought within yourself since thoughts immediately become deeds, and objects immediately materialize. Now it is true that churches are not built there as they are on the physical plane; but let us assume that a being of the astral world wished to realize something, while another sought to prevent it. These things cannot be discussed, but here the principle applies that things must prove their worth! If the two sets of feelers are now present in the same space, they start battling; and then the more fruitful and thus more justified idea—the one that can therefore persist—will destroy the other and be realized. Here, therefore, we have a continual conflict of the most diverse views, thoughts and emotions. On the astral plane, every opinion inevitably becomes deed. Instead of dispute, opinions are left to battle it out themselves, and the more fruitful one will knock the other out of the ring. You can say that the astral world is a much more dangerous one; and some of what is said about such dangers is connected with what I have now described. Everything becomes deed there, and views have to battle with one another rather than discuss and argue.

I will now touch on something that is shocking to hear in our materialistic age but is nevertheless true. We have often stressed that in our era people are increasingly immersing themselves in consciousness of a world that is merely physical, thus also in characteristically physical qualities, distinctive characteristics of the physical world—for instance a world where, in discussion and dispute, each person feels like murdering another who does not share his view or regards him as an idiot. Things are not like that in the astral world. There a being will say: 'Other opinions do not bother me!' The greatest tolerance exists there. If one view proves more fruitful it will knock the others out of the ring. Other opinions can happily exist alongside one's own, since battle will sort it all out. If you gradually come to be at home in the world of spirit you have to learn to judge things according to what is customary there. The first domain of the spiritual world is the astral, where what I have described is customary. Someone who comes to be at home in the spiritual world must, in a sense, make space in himself for the customs of the beings who live there. And this is the right thing to do. Our physical world should increasingly become a reflection of the spiritual world, and we will introduce ever more harmony into our world through accomplishing the following: life in the physical world ought to unfold as it does in the astral world. Although we cannot build two churches in one spot, where views differ we can allow their fruitfulness to interpenetrate in the world. The most fruitful or productive views will be victorious, as is the case in the astral world.

Thus, within a universal spiritual stream, the distinctive qualities of the astral world can really reach down into the physical world. The spiritual-scientific movement has a broad field to cultivate here: to create, increasingly, a reflection of the astral world on the physical plane. However shocking it may sound to people today who only acknowledge the physical plane—and can therefore only conceive of propounding one opinion and seeing anyone who has a different view as a fool—adherents of a spiritual world view will find it increasingly self-evident for absolute inner tolerance of different views to prevail. This is not the sort of tolerance that arises in us like heeding a sermon, but something instead that will take up its natural place in our soul as we increasingly acquire the customs of the higher worlds.

What has been described here, this interpenetrability, is a very important and key quality of the astral world. No being of the astral world will develop a concept of truth such as those we know here in the physical world. The beings of the astral world find debate, argument and so forth to be entirely unproductive. They agree with Goethe that 'Fruitful things alone are true!'[8] We should not come to know truth through theoretical reflections but through their productiveness, through the way in which they prove their value. One being of the astral world will therefore never dispute with another as people do, but will say: Fine, you do your thing, I'll do mine. We will see which is the more productive idea, and which will knock the other out of the ring.

If we engage with this way of thinking, we have already acquired some practical insight. We should not think that our development into the spiritual world is accomplished in a tumultuous way, for actually it occurs subtly. And if we can attend carefully and acquire a quality such as the distinctive characteristic of the astral world I just described, we will increasingly come to regard feelings such as those possessed by astral beings as models for our own. If we allow ourselves to be guided by the character of the astral world, we can be hopeful of living our way upwards towards the spiritual beings whose life, in this way, will become increasingly apparent to us. It is this that will prove fruitful for human beings.

What has been aired today aims in many respects to be a kind of preparation for the subject matter of the next few lectures. We have been speaking of the nature of the astral world and its distinctive characteristics, but we should be aware already that this astral world is far more distinct from higher worlds—say the world of devachan—than people might tend to think. Truly, the astral world is also present wherever our physical world exists. It permeates our physical world, and everything we have spoken of on past occasions always surrounds us, is present in the same space as physical realities and physical beings. But then there is also the world of devachan, which is distinct from the astral world inasmuch as we experience it in a different state of consciousness.

You might easily think that this physical world here is permeated by the astral world, the world of devachan and so on. But things aren't quite so simple as that. If we wish to describe the higher worlds in more detail than we did before, we must be clear that another difference exists between the astral world and the world of devachan. You see, our astral world, in which we live and which penetrates our physical space, is in a sense a dual world, whereas the world of devachan is, in a way, a single world. This is something we needed to mention today as preparation. In a sense there are two astral worlds, and these two differ inasmuch as the first is, as it were, the astral world of goodness while the other is the astral world of evil. It would be incorrect to make such a blunt distinction in the case of the world of devachan. If we consider the worlds in descending sequence we have to see them as follows: first higher devachan, then the lower world of devachan, then the astral world and then the physical world. This does not yet give us the totality of our worlds, for we also have to consider those lower than the physical. Below our physical world there is another, lower astral world. The good astral world lies above the physical plane while the astral world of evil lies below it, and likewise, for all practical purposes, penetrates it. Now the most diverse streams flow into the beings of the astral world. Here we must distinguish between streams of good and bad qualities issuing from human beings. The good streams pass to a good being and the bad streams, correspondingly, connect with a bad being of the astral world. If we take the sum of all good and bad beings of the astral world, in a sense we have two astral worlds. When we observe the world of devachan we will see that this is not true to the same degree. The astral world therefore contains two worlds which interpenetrate and both equally connect with the human being. These two worlds must be distinguished from each other, chiefly in regard to the way they originated.

Looking back to the past evolution of the earth, we come to a time when the earth was still united with sun and moon. At a later period, the earth itself was a moon, a planetary body outside the sun during the old Moon era. At that time an astral world already existed, before our earth became the planet it now is. If this astral world had been able to evolve further without hindrance, it would have become the good astral world. Due to the fact that the moon separated from the earth, however, the evil astral world was incorporated into the general astral world. In our current state on earth we have now reached the point of incorporation of an evil astral world. In future, an evil world will likewise be incorporated into the world of devachan. For the time being let us keep in mind that there are two astral worlds rather than one: into the first enter all the streams that are productive for human progress and evolution; and into the other astral world, to which kamaloka likewise belongs, enter all the streams that inhibit human evolution. In both astral worlds there are entities whose influence on us, and whose mode of coexistence with each other, we have heard about today in a more abstract way. The next time we meet we will consider in more detail the condition and constitution of these beings who populate higher worlds.

LECTURE 2

BERLIN, 21 OCTOBER 1908

In this lecture, which should be regarded as part of the lead-up to our 'annual general meeting campaign',[9] our aim will be to show that spiritual science, or rather the spiritual outlook on the world which underlies it, is in complete harmony and accord with some findings in specific scientific disciplines. As we can see particularly in popular and public lectures, it is not so easy for anthroposophists to meet with full understanding from an entirely unprepared audience. Whenever spiritual science collides with an entirely unprepared audience, the anthroposophist must be somewhat aware that in many respects he speaks a different language from those who have heard nothing at all or only very superficial, external things about insights that underpin the spiritual-scientific movement. It is necessary to delve a little deeper to find harmony and accord between what can so easily be presented in modern science—that is, experiences gained from research into the sensory world—and what is given us through insight gained by means of spiritual, higher, supersensible consciousness. One has to go more deeply into these things before being very gradually able to gain a real overview of this harmony. Then, however, we will see the beautiful harmony existing between what the spiritual researcher asserts and the assertions—that is, the cataloguing of facts—gained through research into physical realities. We should not be too unjust, therefore, towards those who do not understand anthroposophists, since they lack all preparations essential for grasping the findings of spiritual research. In most cases, therefore, they will inevitably conceive both the words and the concepts presented to them in quite different ways than intended. Greater understanding of spiritual science can only be achieved in a broader context, therefore, by speaking from a spiritual perspective, even to an unprepared audience, in an entirely and unashamedly direct way. Then, amongst these unprepared people, there will be a large number who say: 'This is all nonsense, fantasy, gobbledygook!' There will always also be a few, however, whose inmost thirst of soul gives them an intimation that there is, in fact, something behind it; and these people will pursue it further and gradually find their way into it. Such patient delving is the important thing, and this is also what we can aim for. It will therefore be perfectly natural for a large number of those who attend a lecture on spiritual science out of mere curiosity to go away afterwards and spread it about that this is a sect which disseminates its own special brand of codswallop! Knowing these difficulties, though, we can find the necessary calm and patience to countenance the natural process of selection. Members of the audience will find their own path and some will form a core enabling spiritual science gradually to flow into our entire life.

Today I wish to use a particular example to show that well-prepared students of spiritual science, accustomed to thinking and living with the notions which spiritual cognition awakens, can easily relate to the most apparently difficult findings of positive physical and sensory research. The student can gradually acquire a sense that the further he progresses, the more he will see how good a foundation spiritual research provides for all enquiry and insight. This will give the seeker the peace of mind he needs in the face of the tempests which are unleashed against spiritual science because, for many, it speaks an entirely foreign language. And if we have the patience to find our way into this harmony, we will also gain ever greater certainty. When people say, 'What you tell us does not accord with the most elementary scientific research,' then the anthroposophist will reply, 'I know that perfect harmony in relation to all these facts can be established by everything spiritual science can offer, even if at present it may not yet be possible for us to agree.' We will now consider the following, as a special discourse for strengthening awareness in this regard.

When the pupil of spiritual science has lived with a spiritual world-view for a while, he becomes accustomed to speaking of physical body, etheric body and astral body in a way that allows him to make increasing use of these terms, so that they guide and lead him when seeking insight into external things. He must gradually grow accustomed to seeing the physical corporeality surrounding him as differentiated, rather than all of a piece. He looks at a stone but does not say that it is composed of one or another substance like the human body, and that he can therefore treat this body in the same way as a stone. Even the plant, though consisting of the same substances, is something quite different from the stone: it contains both an etheric and a physical body, and would fall apart if it were not entirely pervaded by the ether body. The spiritual scientist therefore says that the plant's physical body would decay if the etheric body did not preserve it from decomposition while it lives, combating this process of decay. If we consider the plant in this way, we find it to be an interweaving of the principle of the physical body and the ether body.

Now I have often stressed that the most fundamental principle of the ether body is that of repetition. An entity solely under the sway of the principle of the ether body and the physical body would manifest the principle of repetition within itself. We can see this in the highest degree in the plant. We can see how it develops leaf after leaf. This is because the physical body of the plant is permeated by an ether body, characterized by the repetition principle: it develops a leaf, then a second, third and so on, adding leaf to leaf in continual repetition. But even when plant growth comes to a stop above, repetition still prevails. At the top of the plant you find again something like a crown of leaves which form the calyx of the flower. These sepals have a different form from other leaves, but you can still become aware that this is only a somewhat altered form of repetition of the same leaves, which ascend in repetition along the whole length of the stalk. Thus we can say that at the top of the plant, too, where it comes to completion, the green sepals are a kind of repetition. And even the petals are a repetition, though naturally they have a different colour. They are still leaves really, though greatly transformed. It was Goethe's great achievement in this field of botany[10] to show that not only are the sepals and petals transformed leaves, but that we should also regard the pistil and stamens as a transformed repetition of the leaves.

But we find more than mere repetition in the plant. If this primary principle of the ether body were the only one at work, the ether body would penetrate the whole plant from below upwards: leaf would follow leaf without end, and the process would never come to completion.

What causes this completion of the plant in the blossom, so that the plant can be fertilized and bring forth a new plant in turn? To the same degree that the plant grows upwards, its astral body comes down to meet it from above, completing and concluding it from without. It brings to completion what the ether body would otherwise continue through eternal repetitions: it brings about the transformation of green leaves into sepals, petals, pistils and stamens. We can therefore say that esoteric insight shows us the plant growing to meet its soul aspect, its astral aspect, and this causes the transformation we observe. The fact that the plant does remain a plant, and does not extend beyond this into voluntary movement or sensation, is because this astral body that comes to meet the plant above does not take inward possession of its organs but only encompasses it from without, working in from above. In so far as the astral body grasps hold of organs within, the plant passes over into the animal. That is the whole difference.

If you think of a flower petal you can say that ether body and astral body work together in it but that the ether body has as it were the upper hand. The astral body is not capable of extending its feeler threads into the plant's interior, but instead only works from without. If we wish to express this spiritually, we can say that what is inward in the animal, what it inwardly experiences as pleasure and sorrow, joy and pain, drive, craving and instinct, is not internal in the plant but continually descends upon it from without. This is certainly a soul-like quality. The animal turns its gaze outwards, takes pleasure in its surroundings, directs its taste perceptions outwards and laps up any enjoyment approaching it from without—thus experiencing pleasure inwardly. Someone who can really observe things spiritually can see that while this astral entity of the plant also has joy and pain, pleasure and suffering, it does so by gazing down upon what it brings about. It takes pleasure in the red colour of the rose and in everything that comes towards it. And when plants develop leaves and flowers, the plant soul looking down on this permeates and tastes it. At that point an exchange occurs between the descending soul part of the flower and the plant itself. In its soul nature, the plant world exists for joy and sometimes also for suffering. Thus we really see a sense of communion between our earth's plant cover and the earth's plant-enveloping astrality, which embodies the plants' soul nature. What works from without as astrality upon plants, engages the animal's soul nature inwardly, thus making it an animal. But there is an important difference between the soul nature active in the astrality of the plant world and in the astrality of animal life.

If you clairvoyantly examine the astrality acting on the earth's plant cover, you find in the soul nature of plants a certain sum of forces; and all these forces working in the plant souls have a certain peculiarity. In speaking of the soul nature of plants, of the astrality which permeates the earth and in which the soul quality of plants unfolds, you must realize that these plant souls in their astrality do not live as do, for example, physical creatures on our earth. Plant souls can interpenetrate so that they flow together as in a fluid element. But one thing is peculiar to them: they develop certain forces, and all of these have the property of streaming towards the centre of the planet. In all plants a force is active that passes from above downwards, seeking the centre of the earth. It is this, specifically, which governs the direction of plant growth. If you extend the axis of plants, you arrive at the earth's centre. This is the direction given by the soul nature descending from above. If we study the soul nature of plants, we find therefore that their most distinctive characteristic is of being penetrated by the rays of forces which all strive towards the earth's centre.

It is different when we consider in general terms the astrality around the earth which belongs to and calls forth animals. Plant soul nature would not as such be able to call forth animal life. To generate animal life, other forces must permeate the astrality. The esoteric researcher who focuses merely on the astral plane can therefore distinguish whether a particular astral substantiality will give rise to plant growth or animal growth. We can distinguish this in the astral sphere. Everything that only manifests forces striving towards the centre of the earth or another planet will generate plant growth. By contrast, forces that stand vertically upon the planet yet also completely and continually circle around it in all directions with exceeding dynamic mobility reveal a different substantiality that gives rise to animal life. Wherever you undertake observations you will find that the earth is wreathed in streams at every location, direction and altitude, and that these form circles around the earth if one extends their direction. This astrality complements the plant astrality extremely well. Both interpenetrate and yet are inwardly distinct. Their inner qualities distinguish them. In other words, at one and the same location on the earth's surface the streams of both types of astrality can interweave. When the clairvoyant examines a particular geographical region, he finds forces that strive solely towards the centre of the earth permeated by others that only circle round it; and then he knows that the latter contain what generates animal life.

I have occasionally emphasized that the astral plane has quite different laws—also different spatial laws—from the physical realm. Tomorrow, when we examine some aspects of four-dimensional space,[11] you will better be able to understand some of what I am now describing in the way of esoteric realities. Today, drawing only on esoteric facts, let us focus on one further peculiarity of this animal astrality.

Taking a physical body, whether plant or animal, we must regard it as something spatially complete in itself; and in a sense we have no additional right to consider something spatially distinct from it as belonging to it. Where physical separation exists, we have to speak of different entities. Only when a spatial or physical connection exists can we speak of a single body. This is not true in the astral world, especially not in the astral sphere which enables animal life to develop. There, astral configurations living separate from each other can constitute a single whole. A particular astral form can exist in a region of space, and another, again spatially complete, can be present in an entirely different part of space. But despite this, these two astral forms, unconnected even by the least spatial thread, can constitute a single entity. In fact, three, four or five such spatially separate configurations can be connected. And the following may even occur. Assume that you have an astral entity of this kind that has not physically incarnated in any way; and then you can find another form that belongs to it. Observing one form you can find something occurring within it which you can call food intake, the consumption of something, because certain substances are being absorbed while others are expelled. And while you perceive this happening in the one form, you can notice that in another, spatially separate astral form, other processes are occurring which entirely correspond to what is happening as food intake in the first. One entity is consuming while the other has a taste experience. And although there is no spatial connection between the two, the process in the one form corresponds fully to that in the other. Thus spatially separate astral forms can indeed belong together. It can even happen that a hundred astral forms, at a great distance from each other, are so dependent on each other that no process can be accomplished without this occurring correspondingly in the others. When these entities then find embodiment in the physical realm, we can discover there reverberations of this distinctive astral quality.

You will have heard, for instance, that twins often show parallel traits that correspond to a remarkable degree. This is because their astral bodies remain related although they are embodied in spatially separate forms. When something occurs in the astral body of one of them, it cannot occur alone but comes to expression also in the astral aspect of the other. Even where it manifests as plant astrality, the astral reveals this distinctive quality of interdependence between spatially entirely separate things. In relation to the plant realm you will have heard of the peculiarity that wine stored in barrels demonstrates a very remarkable process when wine-making time comes round again. The principle which causes the new grapes to ripen is noticeable even in the barrels of wine from a previous year.

I only wanted to mention that visible phenomena always testify to hidden aspects that can be brought to light by methods of esoteric research. From this you can see that it appears quite natural for our whole organism to be astrally composed of principles that are quite different from each other.

There are singular marine animal forms that you can understand if you see them in the context of what we have begun to elaborate here about the secrets of the astral world. In the astral realm, astral forces which mediate food intake do not in the least need to be connected with those which regulate movement or reproduction. When the clairvoyant researcher searches astral space for forms that give rise to animal life, he finds something remarkable: a certain astral substantiality which, when it works within an animal body, he has to see as particularly suited by the forces at work in it to transform the physical into an organ of nutrition. Now quite different astral aspects can exist somewhere which, when they implant themselves in a body, do not form organs of nutrition but instead organs of movement or perception. You can imagine that you have, on the one hand, a system for intake of food while on the other you have one for moving hands and feet. Out of the astral world forces have descended into you but these can stream together from quite different directions. One astral body of energies gives you the one while another gives you the other, and these assemble in your physical body because it has to be a coherent physical form, as dictated by the laws of the physical world. The different bodies of energy assembling from without must there form a single whole. They do not do so from the very outset. We can discover the effect on the physical world of what we have now ascertained through esoteric research in the astral realm.

Certain sea creatures, Siphonophora, lead a very remarkable existence. We find that they have something like a common stem, a sort of tube. At the top of this something develops that really has no other function than to fill with air and then empty again. And this process enables the whole structure to stand upright. If this bell-shaped form were not there, the whole thing attached to it could not remain upright. So this is a kind of balancing system that gives the whole thing equilibrium. This might not strike us as particularly unusual—but we can realize that it is when we see that the upper structure, which gives balance to the whole, cannot survive without nourishment. It is animal by nature, and animals must be fed. Yet it is unable to feed itself since it has no means to do so. In order for this life form to be nourished there are certain outgrowths—quite simply, true polyps—distributed at quite different places on its tube. These polyps would continually tumble over and be unable to retain balance if they were not growing on a common stem. But now they can take up food from without, passing it on to the whole tube that runs through them, thus also nourishing the balancing air system. On the one hand, therefore, we have a system that can only maintain balance, yet on the other also one that can nourish the whole to sustain it. But now we have a life form whose food supply can be very limited: once available food has been ingested, there is nothing left and the creature has to seek out other locations where it can find more food, and for this it requires organs of movement. This is also taken care of, for other structures also grow upon the tube and these can accomplish something different: they do not maintain balance, nor facilitate food intake, but instead have certain muscles which can contract, thus expressing water and so causing a counter-thrust. Thus, once the water has been expelled, the whole structure is impelled in the opposite direction, enabling the creature to reach a food source. Jellyfish propel themselves forwards by expressing water and causing this counter-thrust, and such creatures, which you can say are real movement forms, are also attached here.

In other words, we have here a conglomeration of different animal forms: one type that only maintains balance, then another which only takes care of nourishment, and a third which facilitates movement. But such an entity wouldn't survive at all, would be unable to reproduce, if that's all there was to it. But this is also taken care of. At other places on the tube grow spherical structures whose sole endowment is that of reproduction. Inside these creatures, an interior cavity contains male and female fertilization substances, which fertilize each other there, thus producing more of the species. The business of reproduction is therefore assigned to specific structures in this system which are unable to accomplish anything else.

In addition you find other outgrowths on this shared tube: these are other creatures in which all function has atrophied, and which are only present to provide some degree of protection to what lies below. Here certain life forms have sacrificed themselves, giving up all functions to others, and have become mere covering or surface polyps. As well as this, one can detect long threads, called tentacles, which are again metamorphosed organs. These do not have the functions of the other 'community members', but if the creature is subject to attack from another, they defend it. These are defensive organs. Then there is yet another type of organ, called feelers. These are fine, mobile and very sensitive organs of feeling and touch, a kind of sense organ. The sense of touch that is spread across the whole of our bodies here exists in a specific part.

If we examine things esoterically, what are these Siphonophora you can see swimming about in the sea? Here there is an astral confluence of the most diverse forms: structures for nutrition, movement, reproduction and so forth. And because these diverse virtues of the astral substantiality have sought physical embodiment, they had to thread themselves onto a common substantiality. Thus you see here an entity which in an extremely curious way prefigures the human being for us. If you picture all the organs that appear here in the form of autonomous creatures as connected, interwoven with one another, you have the physical human being, and also the higher animals. Then you can see in a tangible way how realities of the physical world confirm what clairvoyant research tells you: that in the human being, too, the most diverse astral forces stream together and are then held together by the human I; and that when these no longer work together, they allow the human being to break up as a being that no longer feels itself to be a unity, a single whole.

The Gospels speak of numbers of demonic entities that have streamed together and inhabit the human being to form a unity. You will recall that in certain abnormal situations, in cases of mental illness, people lose their inner coherence. There are types of madness where people can no longer keep a grasp of the I, perceiving that their being is sundered into different entities. They confuse themselves with the partial aspects that originally streamed together in the human being.

A certain esoteric principle states that everything existing in the world of spirit will ultimately reveal itself somewhere in the external world. You can see therefore how the conjoined nature of the human astral body is physically embodied in the Siphonophora. Here the occult world peeps through a keyhole into the physical world. If human beings had been unable to wait to acquire sufficient physical density before incarnating, they would be patchwork entities of this kind, though in spiritual not physical form. Size has nothing to do with it. Such a creature, belonging to the coelenterata phylum, beautifully described in every modern treatise on natural history and evoking a kind of rapture in researchers, becomes inwardly comprehensible if we can understand it by considering the esoteric foundations of animal astrality. So here you have an example which can be used when someone speaks to you in a quite different sort of language, saying that physical research contradicts views held in anthroposophy. You can reply that if one is patient enough to correlate these things carefully, even the most complicated of them will turn out to be in harmony. The idea people usually have of evolution is a very simple one, but in fact it did not unfold in such a simple way at all.

To end, I would like to bring up a kind of problem, intended as an assignment; and we will try to solve the problem implicit in it from an esoteric perspective. In studying a relatively low form of animal life we have seen external evidence of an important esoteric truth. Let us now pass to a somewhat higher animal class, for instance the fishes, which can present us with even more riddles. I will only enumerate a few of their characteristics.

We can marvel ever and again at the life of water when observing fish in aquaria. But you should not think for a moment that esoteric insights of any kind might interfere with such studies. If you cast the light of esoteric research findings on such phenomena, and see the other esoterically perceptible entities teeming there to form these creatures as they are, such insight will not decrease but only increase your wonder. But let us consider an ordinary fish—which already offers enormous riddles. The average fish has curious stripes running along its side, also apparent in a different form in the scales. These longitudinal lines run down both sides of the fish, and if you were to rid the creature of these it would start behaving crazily. This is because you would deprive it of its capacity to find the pressure differences in the water—to find where the water buoys it up more, or less, where the water becomes denser or thinner. The fish would then no longer have the capacity to propel itself in accordance with water's pressure differences. Water has different densities in different places, and thus varying pressure is exerted. The fish swims differently on the surface than it does lower down. Through these longitudinal lines fish experience different pressures and all the movements caused by the water's motions. Now the different points on these longitudinal lines are connected via delicate organs—described also in every book on natural history—with the fish's very primitive organ of hearing. And the way in which the fish perceives the movements and inner life of water occurs in a way very similar to that in which we humans register air pressure. It's just that first the pressure conditions exert their influence on the longitudinal lines, and this is transmitted to the auditory organ. The fish hears this. But the whole thing is still more complex: the fish has an air bladder which serves, first, to help it employ the water's pressure conditions and move about within certain states of pressure. The pressure exerted on the air bladder endows the fish firstly with the skill of swimming. But since diverse motions and vibrations act on the air bladder and treat it like a membrane, this works back in turn on the auditory organ, and with its aid the fish orients itself in all its movements. The air bladder is therefore actually a kind of stretched membrane whose vibrations the fish hears. The fish's gills are located where its head ends at the back, and they enable the fish to use the air in the water to breathe.

If you study all these things in the usual biological theories of evolution, you always find that evolution is depicted in a somewhat primitive way. People think that the head of the fish evolves a little more to give rise to the head of a higher animal, and the fins evolve to a somewhat more advanced stage to produce higher animals' locomotor organs and so forth. But things are not that simple if we use spiritual observation to study the processes involved. You see, for a spiritual form that has embodied itself as a fish to evolve to a higher stage, something much more complex must occur. The organs must in many respects be inverted and altered. The forces that act within the fish's air bladder conceal within them, in a kind of matrix or mother substance, the forces which we bear in our lungs. But these are not lost as such. Small parts of them remain but are inverted. In material terms, everything belonging to them disappears, and they then form the human eardrum. In fact the eardrum, an organ that projects outward a good distance in spatial terms, is a piece of that same membrane, and in it are active the forces that once functioned in the fish's air bladder. The fish's gills, furthermore, are reconfigured at least partly into our auditory ossicles, and thus in the human organ of hearing you find transformed gills. Now you can see that it is roughly as if the fish's air bladder had been inverted exactly over the gills. That's why our eardrum is on the outside and the auditory organs lie within. What is entirely external in the fish, those remarkable longitudinal lines by means of which the fish can orientate itself, form the three semicircular canals in us, which enable us to maintain balance. If you were to destroy the three semicircular canals the individual concerned would lose his balance and sense of orientation.

Here we find, instead of the simple process described in natural history, a remarkable astral activity in which inversions continually occur. Imagine that you cover this hand with a glove, but inside it you would have elastic forms. If you now turn the glove inside out, invert it, it will be a very small structure in which the organs that were previously outside become tiny and those that were inside form a broad surface. It is only in this way that we understand evolution—by knowing that inversion occurs within the astral, in the most mysterious way, and that the advance of physical forms arises as though from within this.

LECTURE 3

BERLIN, 23 OCTOBER 1908

In relation to what we call the 'history' of the external physical world, we draw on external documents and reports to trace the previous historical eras of different nations and humanity as a whole. You know of course that by this means, by compiling and studying various documents of more recent date, we can look a long way back to millennia before the birth of Christ. Now you will have gathered from spiritual-scientific lectures that esoteric documents can allow us to look back a great deal further into unlimited realms of the past. Thus we acknowledge an exoteric history relating to the external physical world. And we know that if we speak about the customs, knowledge and general experiences of nations in the centuries immediately preceding our own, about their discoveries and inventions, we inevitably speak in a quite different way than when we go back a millennium or two, and try to describe the customs and habits, the knowledge and insights, of more ancient peoples. History grows ever less familiar as we go back further in time. It might be a good idea to ask whether in fact the words 'history' and 'historical development' only refer to this external physical world, whether events and the physiognomy of the historical process only alter over the course of times so recorded, or whether in fact the word 'history' can also have a meaning when applied to the other aspect of existence, which we describe through spiritual science, and which we pass through in the period between death and a new birth.

Seen in a merely external way to start with, we must acknowledge that our existence in these other worlds, which are supersensible for

modern people, lasts longer than does physical life. So can the word
'history' have any meaning for this world too, for this other aspect of
existence? Or ought we to allow the view that, in the realms in which we
live and through which we pass during the time between death and a
new birth, everything remains the same, constant; that nothing changes
if, for instance, we look back through the eighteenth and seventeenth
centuries to the eighth, seventh and sixth centuries after Christ Jesus
appeared on earth, and still further back into pre-Christian centuries?
Each time we enter upon earthly existence at birth we encounter different conditions on earth. Let us try for a moment to think our way into
the soul of a person—and we are talking of course about our own souls
here—who incarnated in ancient Egypt or ancient Persia. Let us vividly
picture the kinds of circumstances into which someone was born who in
ancient Egypt stood before the gigantic pyramids and obelisks, and
encountered all the customs and conditions we find in ancient Egypt.
Let us picture the conditions that existed in such a life between birth and
death. Now let us imagine that this person dies, undergoing a period
between death and a new birth, and is then born at a period during the
seventh or eighth centuries AD. Let us compare these two epochs. How
very different must the world seem to an incarnated soul in the times
before Christ Jesus appeared here in external form on the physical plane!
Let us continue, and ask: What will be the experience of a soul born,
say, during the first centuries of the post-Christian period, who now
once again enters the physical plane? Such a person will encounter
modern government and national institutions of which there was no
sign in former times. He will experience our modern culture and its
technologies, and in short, such a soul will meet a quite different picture
from the one it encountered in previous incarnations. If we compare
these incarnations, we can see how different they are from each other.
We are therefore entitled, surely, to ask how the circumstances of
someone passing between death and a new birth change and what
happens between two incarnations. A person who formerly lived in
ancient Egypt and then entered the world of spirit after death will have
found particular realities and entities there. Then he enters once more
into physical existence during the first Christian centuries, in turn dying
and passing over again into the other world, and so on. Are we not

entitled to ask whether on the other side of existence, in all the experiences we undergo there, 'history' also unfolds, whether a great many things do not also change there over time?

You know of course that in describing human life between death and a new birth, we give a general picture of its nature. Starting from the moment of death, we describe how, after the great memory tableau has unfolded before a person's soul, he enters upon a period where the drives, desires and passions in the astral body—thus all that still binds him to the physical world—still exist within him, and where what we have become accustomed to calling kamaloka occurs. After shedding these ties he then enters devachan, a world of pure spirit. And we describe what then further unfolds for us during this time between death and a new birth in this purely spiritual existence, until we return once again to the physical world. You have seen how these descriptions have always referred initially to the present time, to our immediate, current life. And this is for good reason. Naturally we have to start somewhere, find a position to occupy, and relate our descriptions to this. Just as we must start with the present when describing present observations and experiences, in accounts of the world of spirit, of the life between death and a new birth, the picture appearing to clairvoyant vision must be described roughly as this unfolds at present for the average person when he dies and, in his passage through the spiritual world, lives towards a new existence. But in the full scope of esoteric observation it becomes apparent that for this world too, which we pass through between death and a new birth, the word 'history' has real significance. Here too development occurs as in the physical world. And just as we give chronological historical accounts of differing events, starting in the fourth millennium before Christ, and trace these through into our post-Christian era, so too, for the other side of existence, we have to acknowledge a 'history'. We become aware that there too, in life between death and new birth, things were not exactly the same in the epochs of Egyptian, ancient Persian or very ancient Indian culture as they are now in our own time. Having formed an initial contemporary picture about life in kamaloka and devachan, it is no doubt time to extend this account and progress to a historical consideration of these worlds. And, to become clear about these things when we present aspects of 'esoteric history', let us be guided immediately by certain spiritual facts. To understand each other, however, we must reach back a long way, roughly into the Atlantean era. By now we can assume that when we speak of those times they are to some degree familiar to each person here.

Let us ask ourselves about the nature of human life beyond the threshold at that epoch, when we can already speak of birth and death. The distinction between life on the other side—to employ a common phrase—and this side of life in the physical world, differed markedly from the distinction we find nowadays. When an Atlantean died, what happened to his soul? It passed over into a state in which it felt entirely secure in a world of spirit, a world of higher spiritual individualities. We know of course that life here in the physical world for the Atlantean was different from our life today. The alternation we are familiar with between being awake and asleep, and unconsciousness during the night was not—as we have often discussed—present in Atlantean times. As a person of those times slumbered over into the other realm, and his awareness withdrew from knowledge of physical things around him, he entered into a spiritual world and perceived spiritual beings. In the same way that we find such things as plants, animals and other people around us during waking life, so in those times a person falling asleep would become aware increasingly, in his sleeping consciousness too, of a world of lower and higher spiritual beings. People lived their way into that world. And when the Atlantean passed over at death into the world beyond, that world of spiritual beings and spiritual occurrences dawned for him all the more clearly and brightly. During Atlantean times people felt their whole consciousness to be far more at home in those higher worlds, those worlds of spiritual occurrences and beings, than in the physical world. And if we go back to the early eras of Atlantis, we find that people then—this was true of all their souls—viewed this physical existence here as a visit to a different world, where they just passed a little time, and felt this realm to be different from their real home, which did not partake of the earthly sphere.

In Atlantean times there was however one peculiarity of life between death and a new birth which it is hard for people today to form an idea about because they have entirely lost it. The capacity to say 'I' of oneself, to feel oneself a self-aware being, to sense oneself as an 'I', which is intrinsic to modern people, was something that the Atlantean lost entirely when he left the physical world. As he ascended into the world of spirit, whether during sleep or to a still greater degree during life between death and a new birth, I consciousness—'I am a self-aware being', 'I am in me'—was replaced by the awareness, 'I am safe within the higher beings', 'I immerse myself in the life of these higher beings themselves.' A person felt himself to be one with the higher beings, and in feeling this merged unity he experienced endless bliss in that realm beyond the physical. His bliss grew ever greater the more he distanced himself from awareness of physical, sensory life. The further we go back in time, the more blissful was this life. And we have often heard of the purpose of humanity's evolution within earthly existence: that human beings should become ever more enmeshed in physical existence on our earth. Whereas the Atlantean felt entirely at home in the other realm in sleep consciousness, experiencing this world as clear, bright and welcoming, on the other hand his consciousness here on earth was still half dreamlike. He did not yet fully take possession of the physical body. When a person awoke, in a sense he forgot the gods and spirits he had experienced in sleep; nevertheless he did not enter physical consciousness on awaking to the degree we do today. Objects did not yet have clear outlines. The Atlantean perceived the world as you may when you go out on a foggy evening and see the street lamps surrounded by a corona, an aureole of all sorts of colours. That is how indistinct all objects of the physical plane were to him. Consciousness of the physical plane was only just dawning, and strong awareness of the 'I am' had not yet taken root in human beings. Only towards the latter days of the Atlantean epoch did human self-awareness, consciousness of personality, increasingly develop in the same degree as blissful consciousness during sleep was lost. The human being gradually conquered the physical world, increasingly learning to use his senses, and so the objects of the physical world also acquired ever clearer and more solid outlines. As the human being mastered the physical world, his conscious awareness in the world of spirit changed.

We have studied the different eras of post-Atlantean times. We have looked back to ancient Indian civilization, seeing how people mastered external reality to the extent of experiencing it as maya, and yearning for the old realms of the land of spirit. We have seen how in the Persian cultural period, conquest of the physical plane had advanced so far already that people wished to connect with the good powers of Ormuzd so as to reshape the forces of the physical world. We also saw how in Egyptian, Babylonian, Chaldean and Assyrian times people discovered in the art of land surveying—which led to agriculture—and also astronomy, the means to advance further in their mastery of the external world. And finally we saw how the Graeco-Roman period went still further, and how in Greece a beautiful marriage arose between the human being and the physical world in the creation of cities or Greek art. Then in the fourth epoch we saw how, for the first time in this form, the personal element emerged in ancient Roman law. Whereas previously the human being felt safely integrated into a whole, as the reflected glory of former spiritual beings, the Roman first felt himself to be a citizen of the earth. The idea of the citizen arose at this time.

The physical world was conquered step by step. But at the same time human beings also came to love it. The human being's inclinations and sympathies united with the physical world. And as sympathy for the physical world grew, human consciousness also merged with physical things. But as this happened, human consciousness grew obscured in the other realm during the time between death and a new birth. That blissful sense of being safely encompassed in the existence of higher spiritual beings was lost in the other realm as human beings came to love this side of life and successively conquer the physical world, as we see from history. Human mastery of the physical world grew by stages: we increasingly discovered natural forces, and invented ever more tools. We came to love this life between birth and death, a process which ran parallel with a darkening of our old, twilight clairvoyance in the world beyond. It never ceased entirely, but it grew more obscure. And as we mastered the physical world, the history of the other world fell into a decline. This decline is related to the rise of a civilization which we describe when we study people who, in the first beginnings of culture, ground their grains between two grindstones, and then advanced stage by stage to make their first discoveries, to procure and learn to use tools, progressing ever further over time. Life on the physical plane became ever richer. Humans learned to construct gigantic buildings.

But in this account of history passing through the Egyptian, Babylonian, Chaldean and Assyrian era to the Graeco-Roman period and thence to our own time we must mark a crucial moment in our account of the advance of cultural history. Balancing this description we must describe a path of decline in the connection between higher gods and what the human being might perform for the gods, what he did on behalf of and within the spiritual world. And we see how in later times the human being increasingly loses his connection with worlds of spirit and with spiritual capacities. We need to write a history of the other realm, too, of human decline there, just as we can write a history of progressive ascent, of ongoing conquest of the physical world for this earthly realm. Thus spiritual world and physical world complement each other, or, more accurately, mutually determine each other.

As you know, this world of spirit interrelates with our physical world. Reference has often been made to the great mediators between the spiritual and the physical world, of the initiates whose souls, although incarnated in a physical body, nevertheless reach up into the world of spirit between birth and death. While human beings are usually quite shut off from the spiritual world during their lifetime, such individuals can experience the spiritual world during their lives and grow accustomed to it. All these messengers—both greater and lesser—of the spiritual world: what importance did they have for human beings? Consider the greatest among them, say the ancient holy Rishis in India, Buddha, Hermes, Zarathustra, Moses or all those who were great messengers of the gods in ancient times. How did all these messengers to us from the gods or from the spirit affect the relationship between the physical and spiritual world?

During, and as a result of, their initiation, they experienced conditions in the spiritual world. Besides seeing with their physical eyes and physical intellect what was occurring here in the physical world, their enhanced capacities of perception also enabled them to experience what was happening in the spiritual world. At the same time as living with others on the physical plane, the initiate can also follow what the dead do in the time between death and a new birth. He is as familiar with them as with people on the physical plane. From this you can see that all accounts of esoteric history in fact flow from initiates' experiences.

An important turning point, also for the history we are now considering, occurred on earth through the appearance of Christ. And we can gain a picture of the advance of history in the other world if we ask what significance the deed of Christ has upon earth. What is the significance of the Mystery of Golgotha for the history of the realm beyond the threshold?

In lectures at various locations[12] I have highlighted the incisive significance of the event of Golgotha for historical developments on the physical plane. But now let us ask how the event of Golgotha appears if we consider it from the perspective of the other side. We can answer this question if we consider the point in evolution in this other realm when human beings had emerged to the greatest degree as citizens of the physical plane, when consciousness of personality had developed most strongly: the Graeco-Roman era. This is also when Christ Jesus appeared on earth. And so we have the most intensively developed sense of personality on the one hand, the most intense pleasure in the sensory world, and on the other hand the strongest, most powerful appeal to the other realm in the event of Golgotha, and the mightiest deed—that of the overcoming of death by life, as embodied in this event of Golgotha. These two things certainly coincide when we consider the physical world. In Greek times there really was great joy in and enhanced sympathy for external existence. Only such people could create those wonderful Greek temples in which the gods themselves lived, as has been described to you. Only such people living in the physical world in *this* way could create those sculptures, which so wonderfully marry spirit with matter; this required pleasure in and sympathy for the physical plane which only slowly evolved through history. We can get a sense of this development if we compare the blossoming of the Greeks in the physical world with the lofty world-view which people in the first post-Atlantean cultures received from their holy Rishis. The latter had no interest in the physical world, feeling themselves at home, instead, in the spiritual world. They looked upward still in bliss to the world of spirit which they sought to reach through the guidance of doctrines and practices given them by the holy Rishis. History travels a long way from this disdain of sensory pleasure to the greatest pleasure in the sense-perceptible world of the Graeco-Roman era, culminating in that marriage between the spirit and the world of senses which accorded both their due.

But what was the counterpart in the spiritual world to this conquest of the physical plane in the Graeco-Roman period? Those who can perceive the world of spirit know that what the Greek poets say of the best representatives of their culture is not merely legend but is based on the truth. How did those who felt themselves entirely within the physical world, entirely sympathetic to it, feel in the world of spirit? When such a figure is given these words, 'Better a beggar in the upper world than a king in the realm of shades!'[13] this certainly corresponds to the truth. In this era the dullest, least vivid state of consciousness arose during the time between death and a new birth. All this sympathy for the physical world went hand-in-hand with a failure to understand existence in the world beyond. It seemed to people as if they had lost everything, and the world of spirit appeared worthless. The more that human sympathy grew for the physical world, the more the Greek heroes felt lost in the world beyond, the world of spirit. Figures like Agamemnon and Achilles felt themselves to be drained or hollowed out there, like empty beings in this world of shades. There were however intervening times—for the connection with the spiritual world was never entirely lost—when such people could live with spiritual beings and spiritual realities. But the state of consciousness I have described was certainly present. Thus we have a decline in the history of the other world that runs parallel to the history of positive progress in this one.

Those we referred to as messengers of the gods or the spirit always had the capacity to pass back and forth from one world to the other. Let us try for a moment to picture what these messengers of the spirit were for people on the physical plane in pre-Christian centuries. Their experiences in the spiritual world enabled them to tell people in ancient times about the real nature of the world of spirit. It is true that they also experienced there the extinguished awareness of physical human beings on earth, but at the same time they perceived the shining wealth of the whole spiritual world. And they were able to bring news to people on earth of the existence of a spiritual world and tell them of its nature and appearance. They were able to bear witness to this world of spirit. This was extremely important in times when human beings increasingly turned their interests outwards to the physical plane. The more people conquered the earth, the greater their joy and sympathy in relation to the physical world, the more also these messengers of the gods had to emphasize the existence of the spiritual world. 'You know various things about the earth,' they could always say, 'but there is also a spiritual world you need to be informed of . . .'—in brief, the messengers of the gods unveiled the whole tableau of the spiritual world to people then. Knowledge of this world was available in various religions. But whenever these messengers of the gods came back down to earth, as it were, after their initiation or after visiting the world of spirit, they were able to bring with them invigoration and elevation from the spiritual world, some of the treasures of the spiritual world, to enrich life on the physical plane that seemed ever lovelier to earthly human beings. Thus they brought the fruits of spiritual life into physical life. What the messengers of the gods brought with them always led people towards the spirit. The world of physical reality, this side of existence, was enriched by the messengers of the gods and the messages they conveyed.

The messengers of the gods could not work fruitfully for the other world to the same degree. The way to think of it is like this. When the initiate, the messenger of the gods, passes over into the other world, the beings there are as much his comrades as are the beings in the physical world. He can speak to them and tell them what is happening in the physical world. But the closer we come to the Graeco-Roman era, the less value there was in what the initiate could offer souls on the other side when he arrived there from the earth, for these souls felt all too keenly the loss of what they had held dear in the physical world. What the initiate could tell them no longer held anything of value for them. In pre-Christian centuries, therefore, the messages initiates were able to bring down to people in the physical world were fruitful to the highest degree, while what they could convey to souls who had departed from the physical world was unfruitful. Buddha, Hermes, Zarathustra brought messages of great import to people in the physical world, but by contrast could scarcely bring much to those in the other world. The messages they brought there were not joyful or enlivening.

Now let us compare what Christ brought about for the world beyond during the Graeco-Roman era—at the time of deepest decadence in the other realm in our esoteric account of history—with what initiates achieved previously. We know the significance of the event of Golgotha for earthly history. We know that it signifies the conquest of earthly death by the life of the spirit, the overcoming of all death throughout earth evolution. We cannot enter into all the details of the significance of the Mystery of Golgotha today, but can summarize it in a few words: it signifies the ultimate, irrevocable proof that life conquers death. And on Golgotha life conquered death, the spirit planted the seed for the ultimate conquest of matter! What the Gospel relates of the 'descent into hell' by Christ after the event of Golgotha, his descent to the underworld of the dead, and his deed there is not a legend or metaphor. Esoteric research will show you that it is true. Just as true as the fact that Christ walked amongst humankind during the last three years of Jesus, so it is true that the dead could rejoice at his arrival among them. Immediately after the event of Golgotha he appeared to the dead, the departed souls. This is an esoteric truth. And now he could tell them that back in the physical world the spirit had irrevocably won victory over matter! This was a plume of light in the world beyond for the departed souls, flaring in a spiritually vibrant way, and reviving the dead Graeco-Roman consciousness of the other realm to initiate a whole new phase for human beings in their life between death and rebirth. Since that time, human consciousness between death and new birth has grown ever brighter.

When we give historical accounts, therefore, we can complement what we say about contemporary conditions with what can be said of kamaloka and life in devachan; and we need to highlight the fact that Christ's appearance on earth marks an entirely new phase for life in the other realm, and that what Christ achieved for earthly evolution comes to expression also in a radical change in the world beyond. This visit of Christ to the other world is hugely significant, and marks a revitalization of life there between death and a new birth. At that important moment of the Graeco-Roman era, departed souls experienced themselves as shadows despite all their pleasure in the physical world, and would therefore have preferred to be beggars in the upper world than

kings in the realm of shades. Since that time, though, they began to feel
ever more at home again in the world beyond. Since then, too, people
have increasingly grown into the world of spirit, so that this moment
marked the beginning of a period of ascent, of blossoming in the
spiritual world.

Though only in brief outline, we have touched on the event of
Golgotha from the point of view of the other world, at the same time
showing that there is just as much a history of the spiritual world as
there is of the physical world. And it is only by studying these real
connections between the physical world and the spiritual world that one
world becomes fruitful for the other in human life. We will repeatedly
see how we gain insight into human life on earth by considering the true
nature of the world of spirit.

LECTURE 4

BERLIN, 26 OCTOBER 1908

TODAY'S lecture aims to explore the conditions that must be met if a person is to develop the powers and capacities slumbering in him, learning to observe higher worlds and acquiring his own experience of them. The articles entitled 'How do we attain knowledge of the higher worlds?'[14] offer a picture of various conditions we need to achieve to pursue the path of knowledge, to penetrate higher worlds. Yet these articles can only present certain aspects, and this would be true even of a series three or even ten times longer, for there is no end to what can be said in this field! It will therefore always be helpful to expand on this theme in one direction or another. In each instance we can only illumine things from a particular perspective; and we should uphold the principle that what has been gained from one angle needs enlarging or extending through insight from another. Today, in brief outline, let us try to cast light from one perspective on some of the conditions of the path of knowledge, conditions for ascending into higher worlds.

You will remember the interpretative suggestions I gave in relation to Goethe's 'fairytale'.[15] Involved here is the fact that we have various kinds of soul capacities and that our ascent depends on the one hand on development of thinking, feeling and will as distinct and separate faculties. At the same time, we need to practise a method that brings these three into the right balance and interrelationship. Will, feeling and thinking must always be developed to precisely the right degree in respect of our specific spiritual goals. For a certain goal, for example, will must hold back while feeling is more strongly accentuated. For another, thinking must take a back seat; and for yet another, feeling. Through esoteric exercises we must develop all these soul faculties in the right proportion, and their development is connected with our ascent into higher worlds.

Above all, it is necessary to cleanse and purify thinking. This is so that thinking shall no longer be dependent on external sensory observation as achieved on the physical plane. As well as thinking, however, feeling and will can also become powers of cognition. They follow individual paths in ordinary life. Sympathy and antipathy are governed by the predilections of each individual. Yet they *can* become objective, cognitive faculties. Scientists today may regard this as inconceivable. It is easy to believe this about thinking, especially when its concepts are geared to sensory observation; but how shall it be acknowledged that feeling can become a source of objective insight if one person feels one way about something, the other another? How could anyone accept that something as volatile and dependent on individual personality as sympathy and antipathy could become a standard for knowledge, and that we could sufficiently discipline them to grasp a thing's inmost nature? It is easy to see that thought does this, but difficult to believe that when we meet an object which awakens a feeling in us such activity of feeling can exist in us in a way that makes it a vehicle of expression for what lives in the object's inmost nature rather than just the individual's own sympathy or antipathy. Likewise, to go further and say that the power of will and desire can become a means to express a thing's inner nature seems at first glance to be downright frivolous.

But in the same way that thinking can be cleansed and thus become objective so that it allows expression of both sensory and higher realities, feeling and will can likewise become objective. Yet we should not misunderstand this: as feeling is ordinarily in people today, in its immediate content, it cannot become the means to express a higher world. This feeling is something personal. The esoteric exercises given to pupils aim to cultivate this faculty of feeling, or in other words to change and transform it. But this makes feeling something different from its former personal mode of expression. When we reach a certain stage on the esoteric path by developing the faculty of feeling as a form of cognition, we should not think, however, that our feeling in relation to an entity before us gives us truth or insight as such. The process is a far subtler and interior one, transforming feeling via esoteric exercises. This is expressed in the fact that someone who has transformed his feelings through such exercises arrives at imaginative perception whereby a spiritual content reveals itself to him in symbols which express realities and entities in the astral world. Feeling changes its nature, becomes Imagination, so that astral images arise in us which express occurrences in astral space. A person perceiving in this way does not see in the same way as in the physical world (for instance a rose overlaid with colours) but instead in symbolic images, and in fact sees in images everything presented to us in esoteric science—the black cross, for instance, decorated with roses. All such symbols seek to express a certain reality and correspond as much to astral realities as anything we see in the external physical world corresponds to physical realities. Thus we develop our feeling faculty, but perceive in Imagination.

The same is true of the will. In reaching the stage that, to a certain level, can be attained by schooling of the will, we do not say when encountering another being that it arouses our appetites but instead, when the will has been developed, we begin to perceive the issuing of sound and tone in devachan.

Feeling is developed in us and the consequence is astral vision in Imagination. The will is developed in us, and this results in experiencing devachanic processes in the spiritual music, the harmony of the spheres, from which the inmost nature of things resounds. Just as we develop thinking and thereby attain objective thinking, the first stage, so the development of feeling leads to the flowering of a new world at the level of Imagination. And in the same way we develop the will whereby perception of the lower devachanic world arises in Inspiration; and finally, in Intuition, the higher devachanic world opens before us.

As we raise ourselves therefore to the next level of existence, images arise which we now no longer apply in the same way as our thoughts, asking how these images relate to reality. Instead, things reveal themselves to us in images composed of colours and forms, and through Imagination we ourselves must unravel the nature of the entities revealed to us in this symbolic form. In Inspiration things speak to us, and we do not need to ask or decipher conceptually, which would be to apply a theory of cognition applicable to the physical plane. No, here the inmost nature of things themselves speaks to us. When we encounter someone who expresses his inmost being to us, this is different from our encounter with a stone. We have to enquire into the stone's nature and reflect upon it. With another human being there is something we do not experience in this way but instead we experience his being in what he says to us: he speaks to us. It is like this with Inspiration. Conceptual, discursive thinking is not at work here but instead we listen in to what things tell us: they themselves give utterance to their nature. It would make no sense to wonder if, when someone dies and I meet him again in devachan, I will know whom I am meeting, since the devachanic beings look different and cannot be compared with what exists on the physical plane. In devachan a being itself says what its nature is, like a person not only telling us his name but also continually letting his essential nature stream towards us. This streams to us through the music of the spheres, and we cannot possibly fail to recognize it.

Now this gives us a certain reference point for answering a question. The diverse spiritual-scientific accounts easily cause misunderstandings, and we can get the idea that the physical, astral and devachanic realms are spatially distinct from each other. But we know that wherever the physical world is, the astral and devachanic worlds are also present, interwoven together. Here we might think that, this being so, we might not be able to distinguish these three worlds as we do in physical space, where everything stands separately. If the realm beyond is interwoven with this realm, how do I distinguish the astral and devachanic worlds from each other? We distinguish them by virtue of the fact that when we rise from the astral to the devachanic plane, tones resonate through the entirety of image and colour forms. What was previously spiritually luminous now begins to resound spiritually. And there is also a difference in our experience of the higher worlds, so that someone who rises up into them can always tell whether he is in this or that world according to particular experiences he has there.

Today I would like to characterize the differences in our experience of the astral and devachanic worlds. It is not only that we can perceive the astral world through Imagination and the devachanic world through

Inspiration, but there are other experiences too that tell us which world we are in.

One aspect of the astral world is the period we pass through immediately after death, called kamaloca in spiritual-scientific literature. What does it mean to be in kamaloca? We have often attempted to describe the nature of this. Frequently I have cited the example of the gourmet ravenous for the experience that only his sense of taste can satisfy. His physical body has been cast off and left behind at death, and to a large degree the ether body likewise, but the astral body is still present. Thus the person remains in possession of the qualities and powers he had during life in the physical body, and these do not immediately alter after death but do so only gradually. If a person has had a longing for tasty food, this longing remains, this appetite for enjoyment—but after death he lacks the instrument to satisfy this since the physical body and its organs are no longer there. He must therefore forego this enjoyment, lusting for something he cannot have. This applies to all kamaloca experiences, which really consist in nothing other than living in the state that obtains in the astral body, having longings for satisfaction that can only be fulfilled by the physical body. Since we do not have this any longer after death, we are obliged to relinquish our search and lusting for such pleasures. This is the period of getting used to doing without them. We are only free of them when we have plucked this longing out of our astral body.

During this whole kamaloca period, what we can call privation lives in the astral body, in the most diverse forms, shades and nuances. This is the content of kamaloca. Just as we can differentiate light into red, yellow, green or blue tones we can likewise differentiate between the most diverse qualities of privation, and this is the quality characteristic of a person in kamaloca. The astral plane is not only kamaloca, however, but is far more wide-reaching. No one who had lived only in the physical world and experienced its content could ever initially experience the other regions of the astral world—whether after death or by other means—without due preparation. Initially, the only way such a person can experience the astral world is through privation.

Someone who rises to higher worlds and knows that he must be deprived of one thing or another, for there is no prospect of receiving it there, experiences the astral world's content of consciousness. Even if someone could by some esoteric means leave his body and gain entrance to the astral plane, he would still have to suffer privation in the astral world.

So how do we develop ourselves so as to become familiar not only with the part of the astral world expressed in privation, the phase of enforced privation, but to experience it in the fullest sense, the part of it which really gives expression to this world in a good sense, in the best sense? By developing the opposite of privation, we can enter the other part of the astral world. Thus methods that awaken powers in us that are the opposite of privation will take us into this other realm of the astral world. These powers must be given us. They are the powers of renunciation. As with privation, many different shades of renunciation are conceivable. The smallest renunciation we undertake takes us a step forward in the sense of developing ourselves upward towards the good aspect of the astral world. By renouncing even the smallest thing, we instil in ourselves something that contributes substantially to our experience of the good aspect of the astral world. This is why so much importance is placed in esoteric traditions on the pupil practising renunciation by renouncing something or other for a while. By doing so he finds admission to the good side of the astral world.

What does such a practice achieve? Let us reflect for a moment on our experiences in kamaloca. Imagine someone passes through death, or by some other means departs from his physical body, so that he lacks the physical instruments of the body and is deprived of all gratification. Privation immediately ensues, and this appears as a pictorial imagination in the astral world. For instance, a red pentagon or a red circle appears. This is nothing other than an image of what enters a person's field of vision, corresponding to the privation in the same way that an object on the physical plane corresponds to our mental picture of it. If a person has very low cravings, primitive desires, gruesome beasts approach him when he emerges from his body. These terrible creatures are the symbol of the lowest cravings. But if he has learned renunciation, then at the moment he leaves his body at death or through initiation, the red circle vanishes because he imbues the red with the feeling of renunciation. It is transformed, and a green circle arises instead. Likewise the animal or creature will vanish through powers of renunciation, to be replaced by a noble form of the astral world.

Through the powers of renunciation we develop through abstinence, we must transform into its opposite what is first given us objectively as the red circle or the hideous animal. From unknown depths, renunciation conjures the true forms of the astral world. No one who wishes to elevate himself to the astral world in a real sense should believe, therefore, that this can be achieved without engaging the powers of his soul. Without this he would only enter one part of the astral world. He must practise abstinence, relinquishing all Imagination also. He who abstains renounces, and this is what conjures forth the true form of the astral world.

In devachan one has Inspiration. Here too an inner distinction exists between its different parts, which we cannot experience passively after death. Less dire things obtain in devachan, due to a certain set of circumstances in the universe. The astral world contains the terrible kamaloca, but devachan does not yet have this. This will only come about in the Jupiter and Venus planetary stages when use of black magic and suchlike will likewise have brought it into a state of decadence. Then of course similar things will develop in devachan as we find today in the astral world. In devachan at the present cycle of evolution, conditions are somewhat different.

What first confronts us when we ascend on the path of knowledge from the astral world to devachan or when we are led upwards on the ordinary path that all of us take at death? What do we experience in devachan? We experience bliss! What differentiates into tones from nuances of colour is certainly bliss. At the current stage of evolution, everything in devachan actively produces and spiritually hears and attunes to knowledge. And here all producing, all hearing of the harmony of the spheres is bliss. In devachan we will feel pure bliss, and nothing but bliss. When we are taken upwards through spiritual knowledge by the leaders of human evolution—the Masters of Wisdom and of the Harmony of Feelings—or as an ordinary person after death, we will always experience bliss in that realm. This is what the initiate will inevitably experience when he has reached this stage on the path of knowledge. But it lies in the nature of the world's progress that it is not sufficient to stop at mere bliss, thus only intensifying the most refined kind of spiritual egotism. The human individuality would then merely continue to absorb the warmth of bliss but the world itself would not progress. If this happened, beings would develop who grew hard within their souls. The salvation and progress of the world therefore requires someone who enters devachan not only to acquire the potential to experience all shades of bliss in the music of the spheres, but also to develop feelings in himself of the opposite of bliss. Just as privation contrasts with renunciation, so the feeling of sacrifice balances bliss—a sacrifice where one is prepared to pour out what one receives as bliss and let it flow forth into the world.

The sense of self-sacrifice was what those divine spirits we call Thrones possessed when they began to play their part in Creation. In pouring out their own substance on Saturn they sacrificed themselves for developing humanity. The matter that exists today is the same that they let stream out on Saturn. And the Spirits of Wisdom likewise sacrificed themselves on ancient Sun. These divine spirits ascended into higher worlds, not only passively receiving the experience of bliss but, in their passage through devachan, learning to sacrifice themselves. They did not grow poorer through this sacrifice but richer. Only a being living entirely in matter believes that he will fade away by sacrificing himself. No, ever higher, richer development is connected with self-sacrifice in the service of universal evolution.

We see therefore that a person ascends to Imagination and Inspiration, and enters the sphere where his whole being is permeated with ever new subtleties of bliss—where, you can say, he experiences everything that surrounds him not only as speaking to him but as an imbibing of the spiritual tones of bliss.

Ascent to higher faculties of cognition involves transformation of all the feelings we have. Esoteric schooling consists in nothing other than the transformation of our feeling and will by practising the rules and methods, tried and tested through millennia, which the Masters of Wisdom and of the Harmony of Feelings have given us. This leads us upward to higher insights and experiences. The pupil will attain these higher faculties by gradual esoteric cultivation and transformation of the content of his feeling and will.

Those who stand within the spiritual-scientific movement should not think it a matter of indifference whether they have belonged to it for three, six or seven years. This means something. The pupil should develop a clear sense of accompanying the inner lawfulness of this inner growth. We must attend to this, otherwise its effects will pass us by.

LECTURE 5

TODAY let us start from simple forms of pain, its primary manifestations. If you cut your finger and sense pain, or bruise your hand or if it is chopped off, the experience of pain involved will be the simplest, most primal kind—and our observations will start here. If we ask modern psychology professionals how they would explain this simplest type of pain, their response nowadays is rather droll. They have made a strange discovery: that pain cannot be explained except by adding a sense of pain to the diverse senses such as smell, sight and hearing. With this, they say, we sense pain, just as we perceive light through the eyes and sounds through the ears. We experience pain because we have a sense of pain, they say. Everyday experience does not give us any grounds for assuming such a thing, yet this does not prevent a scientific outlook founded on pure observation from assuming it. It just goes ahead and invents a sense of pain. Let us not take any further notice of this, however, but instead ask how such a simple, primary pain arises if we cut our finger, and how it is sensed.

The finger is part of the physical body—which contains the substances of the external physical world. Each finger is permeated by the etheric and astral part of the body that belongs to the finger. What is the task of these higher aspects, the etheric and the astral? The physical structure of the finger, composed of carbon, hydrogen, oxygen, nitrogen and so on, these cells assembled in it could not be arranged as they are if the active agent underlying them, the shaper and developer—the ether body—were not present. This originally worked to develop the finger so that its cells came together to compose it, and now also sustains the present composition of cells, preventing the finger from dropping off and decaying. This ether body permeates and fills the whole finger with etheric activity, occupying the same space as the physical finger. But the astral finger is also present. If we have a certain sensation in our finger, a sense of pressure or some other perception, the finger's astral body naturally mediates this, for sensation resides in the astral body.

The connection between the physical, etheric and astral finger is by no means merely mechanical however, but always alive. The etheric finger invariably permeates the physical finger with warmth and strength, continually working to configure its inner parts. What interest does the etheric finger take in the physical finger? It is concerned to put the latter's parts, with whose smallest particles it is connected, in the right place and into the right relationship.

If we now imagine making a small slit in our skin, thus wounding it, this incision will prevent the etheric finger from arranging the finger's different parts in the right way. The ether body is in the finger and seeks to keep the latter's parts together, while the mechanical incision we have made sunders them. Thus the ether finger cannot do what it ought. It is in the same position as we would be if, say, we had made ourselves a tool to use in the garden but someone had broken it. We would then be unable to do the work we had intended, and would be deprived of the chance to do it. This 'being unable' is best summed up by the word 'privation'. And it is this inability to act or intervene that the astral part of the finger experiences as pain.

If we chop off a hand, only the physical hand is chopped off, not the ether hand, and this ether hand is then unable to act any longer. The astral hand experiences this huge deprivation as pain. Thus, in the interplay of the etheric and astral, we acquaint ourselves with the nature of the most primitive, primal pain experiences. This is how pain arises in fact; and it lasts until the astral body has accustomed itself to the fact that this activity is no longer being carried out in this part of the body.

Let us compare this with the experience of pain in kamaloca. There we are suddenly deprived of our whole body; it is no longer present and the ether forces can no longer act. The astral body senses that the whole can no longer be organized and it yearns for the activity that can only be carried out by means of the physical body, experiencing this privation as pain. Every experience of pain is a suppressed activity. Every suppressed activity in the cosmos leads to pain and, since activity must frequently be suppressed in the cosmos, pain is something necessary there.

However, something else can occur. Through privation processes and suchlike the hand can to a certain degree be [held back] from its distinctive, vital activity, so that its functions are suppressed. This is the case, for instance, if a person starts to scourge or chastise himself, thus bringing bodily organs that were formerly in full, lively activity to a certain standstill. Then, in the case of the hand for instance, the astral part withdraws from the ether hand. The latter then has an excess of forces: it has lost its mission despite still having the capacity to engage in its usual activity. Despite suffering no actual wound, it has lost its purpose. If a person does this, he starts to sense excess powers in the astral body and recognizes the availability of these excess powers. 'Previously,' he will say, 'I used all my strength in regulating the physical body, but now I have constrained and tamed it.' In doing this and no longer using up so much strength or energy, the astral body will feel these excess forces as bliss. You see, just as suppressed activity causes pain, so accumulated strength gives a sense of bliss. The astral body's capacity to do more than it was inherently predisposed to do means bliss for it. This awareness of brimming energy, which can rise up in producing what is available to be governed from within outwards since it is not used by the external body, signifies bliss.

What is the purpose of scourging the physical body, as this is practised in monastic orders? What does this mean? Here less use is made of the functions of the physical body, which are thus quietened so that some capacity is retained in the etheric body. Let us picture firstly a person who has lived in self-imposed privation and who has gradually succeeded in making his physical metabolism act calmly and quietly without calling upon the ether body much; and then someone who likes to eat as much as he can, in a chaotic fashion, engaging his digestion at full tilt. In the person who undertakes everything placidly, whose physical functions may even show some sluggishness and do not call so much on the forces of the etheric body, the ether body retains certain powers. The other person, by contrast, must use up all his etheric forces to sustain his physical functions. In consequence the person who has quietened his body and reined in its appetites possesses excess forces in his etheric body, and the astral body mirrors this as powers of cognition—not merely bliss—so that such a person can perceive imaginative pictures of the astral world. Savonarola,[16] for instance, had a physical body that did not much tax him: he was frail, even continually a little sick, having much in his ether body that could not be used up by being directed into his physical body. He could therefore use these powers to access his mightily powerful thoughts and impulses, giving potent speeches which inspired his listeners. The visions he also had enabled him to present to his audience mighty prophetic pictures.

And now we can apply this to the spiritual worlds. Just as inhibited activity is privation in kamaloca—and privation is *the* kamaloca state— when we enter devachan all suppressed activity falls away because nothing remains there that is in any way connected with the physical plane or yearns back hungrily for physical things. Here we are given up to spiritual substantiality, which gradually builds up the form of our next incarnation. Here is the purest, most uninhibited activity, which we experience as the purest bliss. In life we continually learn from everything that surrounds us. The bodies, though, which we have now, are ones we built up in accordance with the powers of our former incarnations: we have built them up through these powers. What we encounter and acquaint ourselves with in this life is not yet in our body. During our life we change: our feelings and emotions change, our ideals grow. A great sum of inhibited urge for activity sits in us but we cannot transform our body. We have to make do with it as it was built up in line with the experiences of former incarnations. In devachan we are liberated from these constraints and in consequence our unconstrained urge for activity lives its life to the full in bliss. There we create our astral body, etheric body and physical body for the next life. What remains unused here on earth is integrated in devachan. We bear with us up to devachan not only our present, modern consciousness, but also what exceeds the scope of our personality, and this gives us an elevated existence there. In addition to the nature of our individuality here we also experience in devachan what we have acquired to enhance it, the accomplishments added to it, but were not yet able to bring to expression during our lifetime. In this way we can understand all stages passing from the lowest level of pain and privation right up to bliss. In one world we can always trace the signs of what threads through all worlds.

Today therefore we can also better evaluate the ascetic methods developed through history. Just as pain is connected with external injuries to the physical body, so a sense of bliss is connected with a decrease in outer and thus an enhancement of inner activity. This is the sensible aspect of old forms of asceticism, and we can understand why, through renunciation, people have sought a path leading up to higher worlds. Often we have to be clear about the most primitive aspects in order to grasp, in a sense, how spiritual science can explain the path leading from privation and renunciation to bliss through something as simple as a finger injury; and likewise how bearing bodily pain can become a kind of path of knowledge. Everything is semblance and resemblance,* and if we explain the small thing we see in front of us as spiritual science reveals it to be, we gradually elevate ourselves to a spiritual height that will enable us to understand the loftiest things.

If we compare this with what we spoke of yesterday, we can see why bearing bodily pain can be a kind of schooling, a path of knowledge. Think of a person who has never had a headache. He might say that he is unaware of having a brain since he has never felt it. And then let us consider that such a headache does not come about due to external influences but arises at a certain stage of Christian initiation, referred to as the 'crowning with thorns'. Here a person has the sense that whatever sufferings, pain and constraints approach him, seeking to undermine what is most important to him, his mission, he will stand upright even if he has to bear it alone! If someone were to practise cultivating these feelings for months, indeed for years, he would ultimately arrive at the feeling of such a headache, as if thorns were piercing his head. This is a transition towards perceiving the esoteric forces that formed the brain. When the brain's etheric forces do precisely what they must, they find nothing that could bring these forces to our awareness. But the moment

---

* Translator's note: This refers to a phrase in Goethe's *Faust* 'Alles vergängliche ist nur ein Gleichnis,' which could be translated as 'Everything transient is but a semblance.'

the physical brain is in a sense wounded under the influence of these feelings, the etheric body must detach itself, must withdraw from the brain, is driven out of it, and this independence of the etheric head leads to knowledge and insight. This transitory pain is only a transition towards attaining powers of cognition, involving nothing other than objectivizing what we did not previously know. A person may not previously have known that he had a brain, but now he learns to perceive the etheric forces and their activity which have built up and sustain his brain.

There are various other things that could be said. When a physical organ is separated from its etheric element so that the latter cannot intervene, we feel pain. Once the astral body has accustomed itself to this, healing or scarring occurs as liberation of the etheric body, so that, in other words, not all the forces of the etheric body are used. Then the reverse occurs: a feeling of joy and bliss.

LECTURE 6

BERLIN, 29 OCTOBER 1908

Today we will consider things you are already familiar with from a certain angle.[17] All spiritual-scientific studies, however, can only be fully illumined when we shed light on them from a range of different perspectives. In the anthroposophical stream here in our Central European regions we need to discuss certain things, drawn from advanced esoteric research, which could therefore easily be misunderstood. At the same time we would make no headway without taking the risk of talking about them in a quite unvarnished fashion.

In retracing humanity's evolution through the different periods of civilization in the post-Atlantean period back to Atlantis, and further back to still more ancient times, we find, when we focus a spiritual gaze on the processes involved, that the human being assumes ever-changing forms. In the last third of the Atlantean epoch, the etheric body was still outside the physical body to some extent. The head of the etheric body was not yet connected with the powers of the physical body—which are the forces of the I, of self-awareness. If we observe the process underlying this, we find that further evolution involved the etheric head pushing its way into the physical head. If you look at a horse today, its etheric head extends well beyond the physical head. Compared with the physical head it is a mighty form. I have also described to you the magnificent organization of an elephant's etheric parts, which extend way beyond its physical body. In the same way, in the Atlantean period, the human etheric body was outside him, and only gradually penetrated. This kind of penetration by a thinner element of a denser one at the same time involves what is physical becoming more compact. In those times, therefore, the physical human head had a quite different appearance from later on.

If we were to look still further back, to the latter days of the Lemurian epoch, a spiritual gaze would see very few signs of the physical head, which existed then only in very soft, transparent matter. Only through gradual penetration by the etheric head did parts of the head become denser and separate from parts of the surrounding world. In later Atlantis, too, people were still hugely endowed with something that is only retained now in the pathological state of hydrocephalus, or water on the brain. We must also picture the bones of the upper human limbs in a softened state, completely soft. This sounds terrible to people today. Out of this watery substance has hardened and formed what today encloses the human head. The image I sometimes use, of a salt solution in a glass hardening and crystallizing out of water, is not far removed from what happened. The way salt crystallizes out of a watery solution reflects these things fairly accurately. What occurred with the human head at this late stage happened to the rest of the human being much earlier. The other limbs also gradually evolved from a soft mass.

We can therefore ask where the human I was at that time, the I of today. It was not really in the human being, but still in the surrounding world. As the I entered, we can say too, the upper human limbs hardened. The fact that the I was still outside us then endowed it in another respect with a quality that later changed. By increasingly coming to dwell in the physical body, the I was obliged to become an individual I, whereas previously it was still a kind of group soul. Let me give you an image for this state of affairs. Imagine twelve people sitting in a circle somewhere. The stage of evolution we have reached today means that each of these has his I within him. You can say therefore that there are twelve I's sitting in the circle. But if we observed such a circle in Atlantean times, while the physical bodies would likewise be sitting around, the I would still be outside in the ether body. In other words, each person would have his I in front of him. But the I had another quality then: it was not so centralized, it immediately activated its powers and connected with the I's of the other people. Here, therefore, they form a ring that in turn sends its forces back towards the centre.

Thus we have an encircling etheric body here forming a single whole, and enclosed within it the I's. This image, of a circle of physical bodies, then an etheric ring inside it forming a unity that results from every individual I enclosed within it, can give us a tangible idea of group souls.

If we go still further back, we can retain this image but must no longer conceive of such a regular circle of people. Instead they may be scattered across the world. We can imagine someone in western France, another in eastern America and so on, thus not sitting together but, as far as the laws of the spiritual world are concerned, the I's can be together even if the people are scattered across the globe. These people are then interlaced. What is formed then by the confluence of their I's is not such a geometrically beautiful ether body but is still a unified entity. Thus at that time a united group of people existed by virtue of their I's forming a unity; and there were really four such group I's. You have to picture these people in accordance with the laws of the spiritual world. The group souls of the four groups interwove with each other; they were not inwardly united but entered into each other. These four group souls are called by the names of the four creatures of the Apocalypse, eagle, lion, bull and man. But the human being was then at another level of evolution from today. These names derive from the organization of the group souls. How did they come to be called by these names? Today I would like to explain this to you from another angle.

Let us transport ourselves back for a moment to gain a vivid sense of the early era of Lemuria. The souls incarnated today in human bodies had not yet descended as far as to enter physical bodies; as yet they had no inclination at all to unite with physical matter. The bodies, too, that would later become human bodies still very closely resembled animals. On earth we find grotesque physical entities that would appear more grotesque even than the most grotesque creatures on earth today. Everything, both human beings and their environment, was still in a state of soft, slippery matter, either watery or bubbling fire. Amongst these grotesque forms, of course, the antecedents of the human physical body were present, but the I had not taken possession of them. The four group souls we described were already living as four group souls before the spirit entered the human physical organization; and thus four I's were awaiting embodiment—I's inherently disposed towards very specific forms to be found below. Some had the predisposition to be drawn to one kind of organization already present in quite specific physical forms, and others to other such organizations. The shapes of the life forms below had to correspond in a certain way to the nature of each I that was waiting there. Some forms were particularly suited to receiving the lion I, others the bull I and so forth. This was at a very early stage of earth evolution. Now picture the group soul which we have called the bull soul drawing towards very particular forms below. These have a specific appearance; and likewise the lion soul was drawn towards particular forms.

Thus physical nature on earth reveals a fourfold image. One group evolved organs in particular whose functions correlated more with those of the heart—their organization was one-sidedly oriented to the heart. They bore within them an especially aggressive, courageous, attacking element. Full of courage, they wished to dominate and overcome the others; so you can say they were already conquerors by nature, and this was implicit in their form. These were entities in whom the heart was made strong as the seat of the I. In others the organs of digestion, nutrition and reproduction were most developed, while in a third group the organs of movement were emphasized. In a fourth group all these elements were distributed in equal measure, so that the element of aggression and courage was balanced by the calm element that enters through development of the digestive organs. The group in which the aggressive element was most developed, associated with the heart organization, were the human beings whose group souls belonged to the lions. The second group was that of the bull; the third group, with the element of movement that does not care to know much about earthly things, belonged to the group soul of the eagle. These were the ones who could raise themselves above the earth. And those in whom all these things were in equilibrium belonged to the group soul 'man'. In the physical realm, therefore, we discover a projection of these four group souls.

In those times the observer would have seen a quite remarkable sight. He would have found a sort of race which, with prophetic knowledge, he could have identified as physical beings reminiscent of lions, reflecting lion character, despite looking different from today's lions.

These were lion-hearted entities, aggressive precursors of human beings. Then again there was a group of bull-like entities, all as considered from the physical plane. You can easily deduce the third and fourth race for yourselves. The third was already strongly visionary in nature. Whereas the first loved to battle and the second cultivated everything connected with the physical plane and its assimilation, the third class of humans you would have found to be very visionary. On the whole they had something that looked deformed in relation to the other bodies. They would have reminded you of people who have great psychic gifts and believe in visions but who, since they do not pay much attention to the physical realm, have a somewhat desiccated quality, something atrophied by comparison with the burgeoning strength and energy of the other two groups. They would have reminded you of bird nature. These eagle-men tended to want to 'hold back' or retain their spirit. The others had something that was composed as it were of all aspects.

Something else must be considered. If we go far enough back to find such conditions on earth, we must also keep in mind that everything that had happened during the earth's evolution occurred so that the spirit could regulate earthly affairs. All this was simply a detour to arrive at the modern human being. Anyone who could have examined these things still more closely would have found that these lion natures, reminiscent of what we see today in a quite different way in the form of the lion body, developed a special power of attraction for the male forms of ether bodies. They felt themselves especially drawn towards these lion men, and thus these beings had an outward lion body but an inner masculine ether body. Such a creature was a mighty ether being, masculine in character; and a small part of this ether being consolidated into the physical lion body. You can really say that the physical body was the comet nucleus while the ether body formed the comet's tail, as the real creator of the nucleus. The bull race, however, had a special power of attraction for the feminine ether body. Thus the body of the bull creature had the power to attract the feminine ether body and unite with it. And now imagine, also, that the effect of this is ongoing, and that the ether bodies continually penetrate and transform the physical.

The relationship between the lion-type and bull-type person is particularly important in ancient times. The others are less relevant. The masculine ether bodies, which crystallized a physical lion body out of themselves, had the capacity to fertilize the physical lion body itself; and thus reproduction of humanity was ensured by the lion-type race. This was a kind of non-sexual fertilization proceeding from the spiritual realm. The bull-type race was also able to do this. What had become physical worked back here on the feminine ether body. During the course of evolution things started to change. Whereas the lion nature preserved this kind of reproduction, and intensified it, since the fertilizing power descended from the spirit from above, the other process was increasingly suppressed. Bull humanity grew ever less fertile. In consequence, one type of humanity was sustained through fertilization while the other half became less and less fertile. One type became the female sex and the other the male. What is today physically female in fact has a male ether body while the man's ether body is feminine. The woman's physical body emerged from lion nature while the physical bull body is the precursor of the male body.

The spiritual nature in us has a common origin, is neutral, only entering the physical body after the sexes had already become differentiated. Only then was the spiritual element taken up, and only then did the head harden. Not until this point did the ether body of the head unite with the physical body, entirely unconcerned as to whether it settled on the body of a man or a woman. Both sexes are the same in this respect. Ignoring the general commonality over and above sexual differentiation, we can say that the woman has evolved something lion-like. We can certainly discover this concealed courageous aspect in her. The woman can develop the courage of inwardness in war for example, in nursing, in certain services to humanity. The male physical body has what we can really call bull nature. This is connected with the man's greater tendency to act out of physical endeavour. This is certainly apparent from an esoteric perspective, even though it sounds very odd. Thus you see how these group souls have acted together. They work in collaboration, the lion and the bull group souls. These divine entities act together, and today we can find within us the labours undertaken by the diverse divine group souls.

The images I have briefly offered here can certainly take effect. In tracing humanity back to ever earlier times, until we reach an era when reproduction was not yet possible, we must say that the external physical female body transformed into something lion-like whereas the male body was bull-like. If we wish to understand these things properly, we must approach them only with reverent, serious respect. Students of human anatomy would find it easy to derive the anatomical divergences between man and woman from the different natures of lion and bull. As long as physical scientists study only external facts instead of penetrating into inner spiritual realities, their work will remain entirely unproductive.

Now it will no longer strike you as so strange that a former race of humans once had lion-like bodies. These increasingly incorporated the nature of the I so that lion nature was transformed ever more into the female body. Those which did not integrate anything of this spiritual element transformed in a different way—into the actual lions of today and what is related to them. On another occasion I will explain why these animals also have two sexes. Those which did not gain any of this spirituality evolved into today's lions while those that did developed today's female body.

Over time, we can demonstrate a very great number of other related aspects. Anthroposophic study is not like mathematics. First we draw attention, for example, to the four group souls, initially only naming them. Then we choose a particular point of view, and illumine the matter from without. And so we keep approaching things from different perspectives. We circle round the original premise and illumine it from the most diverse points of view. If you take this on board, you will never be able to say that anthroposophical findings are contradictory. The same applies even to the greatest things we consider here. The apparent contradictions are due to the different standpoints we adopt in our studies.

I would like to think that you will take what one might call inner tolerance away with you. May we succeed in introducing this inner spirit of tolerance into our distinctive anthroposophic stream, the anthroposophic movement. Let us take this away with us as a content of our feeling, and try to work in the wider world in a way that can allow this spirit of profound, inmost mutual understanding to take root. Even if we are in different locations, our soul, our heart can reach out to all that unites us, to the great anthroposophical ideals. And then we can elaborate what a spiritual organism should be, as something that grows and thrives: the life of our anthroposophic cause towards which we send our strength from the most diverse angles and perspectives.

LECTURE 7

BERLIN, 2 NOVEMBER 1908

TODAY we will embark on spiritual-scientific studies that show us
how the knowledge we acquire through the anthroposophic world-view
can give us insights into life in the broadest sense. Besides developing
greater understanding of mundane reality through such knowledge, we
also gain broad, wide-ranging insights as we trace life beyond death into
the time unfolding for us then between death and a new birth. But
spiritual science can be of great benefit precisely for ordinary daily life,
solving various riddles and showing us how, if you like, we can cope
with life. For those whose gaze cannot delve into the foundations of
existence, much of what they encounter in life on a daily, indeed an
hourly basis will be incomprehensible. Many questions will build up for
them, which sensory experience cannot answer but which, if they remain
unresolved riddles, can disrupt life by causing dissatisfaction. Dissatisfaction in life, however, can never lead people further or serve
humanity's real salvation. There are hundreds of riddles of this kind
which we could consider, and which illumine life in a much more
profound way than we might expect.

The word 'forget' is one that conceals many mysteries; it of course
designates the opposite of retention of a particular idea, thought or
impression. No doubt you have all had some dismal experience of what
this word represents. You have probably all suffered the agony of being
unable to recall some idea or impression because it has vanished from
your memory. You may then also have wondered why forgetting has to
form part of our experience of life.

Only insight into esoteric realities can help us understand such a thing. As you know, memory or recall is connected with what we call the human etheric body. We can therefore assume that the opposite of remembering—forgetting—will likewise have something to do with the etheric body. It may be justified to ask whether any purpose is served by the fact that we can forget things we have once had in our mind. Or must we instead—as so often happens—accept the negative characterization of forgetting as a deficiency of the human soul, our inability to keep everything in mind at once? We will only gain insight into forgetting if we call to mind the significance of its opposite, the importance and nature of memory.

When we say that memory is connected with the etheric body, we also have to ask why it acquires this role of retaining impressions and ideas. After all, a plant has an ether body, and there it has a substantially different function. We have often discussed the fact that in contrast to a mere stone the whole materiality of a plant we see before us is permeated by its ether body. In the plant the ether body is the principle of life in the strict sense, and then also that of repetition. If a plant were subject only to the activity of the ether body, then the leaf principle would simply keep repeating from the root upwards. It is due to the ether body that parts of a living entity keep replicating anew, for it always seeks to keep producing the same thing. Something like this also occurs of course in reproduction, the producing of one's own species, and this is largely dependent on the ether body's activity. Everything in us and in animals that depends on replication can be ascribed to the etheric principle. The fact that vertebrae keep repeating in the spine is due to this activity of the ether body. But where all the plant's vegetative growth culminates in the flower, this is due to the earth's astrality descending into the plant from without.

The human astral body is likewise responsible for the way the vertebrae expand as they rise to form the skull, becoming hollow. We can therefore say that whatever induces completion and conclusion is subject to the astral body while all recapitulation derives from the ether body. The plant has this ether body, as we do also. Of course a plant has no memory. To claim that a plant has some kind of unconscious memory that induces it to take note of the nature of the leaf it has produced, before continuing to grow a little and then repeat the pattern by putting forth another leaf, takes us into the kind of fantastical territory to which modern scientists have recently given credence.[18] People say, for instance, that heredity derives from a kind of unconscious memory. Currently this has led to some nonsensical notions in scientific literature, for the plant has no memory, and to say that it has is really just amateurish in the extreme.

The etheric body here enacts the principle of recapitulation. To understand the difference between the ether body of the plant and that of the human being, which in addition to the functions of the plant's ether body also has the capacity to develop memory, we have to clarify how plant and human being differ overall. If you imagine planting a seed in the ground, a quite specific plant will grow from it. A wheat grain will produce a wheat stalk and ears of wheat, whereas a bean will produce a bean plant. The way a plant develops is unalterably deter-mined in a specific way by the nature of the seed. While it is true that a gardener can come along and enhance or reshape the plant by all sorts of horticultural methods, basically this is just a sort of exception to the rule, and is also very limited in scope compared with the general principle we stated: that a plant developing from its seed will assume a very particular form, and grow in a very specific way and so on. Is the same true of us? Certainly, to a certain degree—but only so far. When a person emerges from the human seed we see that he is subject to certain developmental strictures: a black child is born to black parents, a white child to white ones. We could give various examples here to show that the growth of human beings, like that of plants, occurs within certain limitations. But this holds true only within certain parameters, within the confines of physical, etheric and also astral nature. A child's habits and inclinations, which remain with him throughout life, can be shown to resemble passions and instincts of his ancestors. But if we were confined within the limits of a certain kind of growth as the plant is, there could be no such thing as education or the unfolding of qualities of soul and spirit.

Think of two different sets of parents giving birth to two children whose disposition and outward characteristics resemble each other closely; and then imagine one of the children being neglected, with scarcely any attention paid to educating him, while the other is conscientiously educated, sent to a good school and helped to develop fully. You cannot say that rich development of this kind was present in the seed of the child already as, say, in the bean. The bean plant will grow whatever happens, and does not need to be educated—that's its nature. We cannot educate a plant, but we can educate children. We can pass things on to the child, introduce him to things, whereas the plant is immune from such efforts. What is this due to? It is due to the fact that in every instance the plant's ether body possesses a certain intrinsic lawfulness, closed off from outer influence and developing from seed to seed: a certain scope that cannot be exceeded. The human ether body is different. Besides the part of it used for growth, for the same kind of development that in a sense encompasses us as it does the plant, there is another part of the ether body, you can say, that exists freely and has no prior use unless we teach the child all sorts of things in educating him, incorporating into the human soul all manner of things which this free part of the ether body makes use of and assimilates. In other words, there really is a part of the human ether body in us that nature does not use. We retain this and do not use it for growth, do not apply it to natural, biological development, but retain it within us as something intrinsically free by means of which we can assimilate the ideas and images which approach us through education.

This assimilation of ideas occurs initially however by virtue of the fact that we receive impressions. We must always receive impressions since all education is also based on impressions and on collaboration between the etheric and astral bodies. To receive impressions, you see, we need the astral body. But to retain an impression so that it does not fade again, the etheric body is needed. The activity of the ether body is necessary for retaining even the least, apparently most insignificant memory. For instance, if you look at something, you need the astral body. But to retain it after turning your head away, you need the etheric body. The astral body is involved in looking at things, but the etheric body is necessary for retaining the image of it. Though very limited activity of the etheric body retains images in this way, and though it really only comes into its own in relation to lasting habits, inclinations, changes to temperament and so on, nevertheless, this is where it is needed. To retain even a simple idea in our head the etheric body has to be present, since all retention of ideas is in a sense based on memory.

Through educative impressions, through mental development, we incorporate all kinds of things into the free part of our etheric body, and must now ask whether this free part remains of no importance whatever for growth and development. That is not so. The older we become—not so much in younger years—all the educative impressions incorporated into our etheric body participate in the whole life of the human body, also inwardly. You can best understand the nature of this participation if I tell you something that is not usually considered in ordinary life. People think that soul qualities generally have little significance for human life. But the following can happen: someone falls ill simply because he has been exposed to adverse climatic conditions. Now we have to picture hypothetically that he can be ill under two types of condition: firstly in a state where he does not have much to assimilate in the free part of his ether body. Let's assume that he is lethargic, and the outer world makes little impression on him, that he has put great obstacles in the way of educational efforts in his direction—that things have gone in one ear and out the other. A person like this will not have the same means of recovery as someone else who possesses a lively, active sensibility and has absorbed a great deal in his youth, assimilated a great deal, thus taking very good care of the free part of his ether body.

Practitioners of mainstream medicine, of course, still have a way to go before they can ascertain why greater obstacles to the process of recovery are apparent in one person than in the other. This free part of the ether body, in which manifold impressions have engendered dynamism, comes to the fore here and its inner mobility participates in the process of recovery. In numerous instances people owe their rapid or painless recovery to the fact that, in their youth, they diligently assimilated the impressions offered to them. Here you see the effect of the spirit on the body! Trying to cure someone who passes through life with dull sensibility is a very different matter from doing the same for someone whose free part of the ether body is not sluggish and lethargic, but has remained active. Empirical evidence of this can be ascertained simply by observing the world with open eyes and seeing the different ways in which mentally lazy and mentally active people respond to illness.

So you can see that the ether body is something quite different in people than in plants. The plant lacks this free aspect of the ether body which allows us to develop. Basically all human development depends on us having this free aspect. If you compare the beans of a millennia ago with those of today, you will see that the difference between them—though there is one—will be very small, and that basically they have remained the same. But compare Europeans at the time of Charlemagne with Europeans today. Why do people today have very different ideas and feelings? It is because they have always possessed a free aspect of their ether body which enabled them to assimilate things and transform their nature. This is all true in general. But now let us consider how all that we have described actually functions in detail.

Let us take the example of someone who, having received an impression, is unable to erase it from his memory again. It would be a strange thing to imagine that everything that has ever made an impression on you from childhood on should be present in your mind every day of your life, from morning through to evening. As you know, all this is only present to your awareness for a certain period after death, where it serves its proper purpose. But during life we forget things. All of you have not only forgotten countless things that you experienced in childhood, but also a great deal of what happened to you last year, and no doubt also some of what happened yesterday. A notion that has disappeared from your memory, which you have 'forgotten', has not however vanished from your entire spiritual organism, the record and pattern of your being. This certainly isn't the case. If you saw a rose yesterday and have now forgotten it, the image of the rose is still present in you, as are all the other impressions you absorbed—even if they have been forgotten as far as your immediate awareness is concerned.

Now there is really an enormous difference between an idea or picture while you remember it and the same idea when it has disappeared from your memory. So let us consider an image formed in response to an external impression, which is now living in our awareness. Then let us cast our eye of soul on the way it gradually disappears, is gradually forgotten. It is still present though within our whole spiritual organism. What is it doing there? What is this 'forgotten image' preoccupied with? It has its own very important role. You see, it only begins to work upon this free part of the ether body which I described, and to render this free part of the ether body of use to us once it has been forgotten. It is as if this image or idea has only then been properly assimilated. As long as we make use of it in order to know something with its aid, it is not working inwardly on the free mobility, on the organization of the free part of the ether body. The moment it fades and is forgotten it starts to work. And so we can say that ongoing work is continually underway within the free part of our etheric body. And what is it that undertakes this work? The labourers are our forgotten ideas. That is the great blessing of forgetting! As long as an idea or image sticks in your mind, you relate it to an object. If you observe a rose and retain the memory of it, you relate the rose image to the external rose, so that the image is bound to the external object and is obliged to send out its inner energy towards it. But the moment you forget the image, it is inwardly released and starts to develop germinal powers that work inwardly upon your etheric body. Our forgotten notions therefore have major significance for us. A plant cannot forget nor, of course, can it receive impressions. Simply because it uses up all its ether body for the purposes of growth it would be unable to forget, since there is no unused remainder. Even if ideas could enter it, a plant would have nothing with which to develop them.

But everything that happens does so in lawful necessity. Wherever something is present that needs to develop but is not supported in its development, an obstacle to development is created. Everything in an organism that is not incorporated into development becomes a hindrance to development. If all kinds of occlusions were secreted within the eye, substances that could not be assimilated into its general aqueous nature, vision would be impaired. Nothing may remain that is not integrated and absorbed. The same is true of mental impressions. Someone who, say, could receive impressions but had to retain them continually in his mind, would soon be likely to reach a point where the part of the ether body that should be nourished by forgotten notions would receive too little of such sustenance and would then hamper development like a paralysed limb instead of furthering it. This is also why it is injurious for someone to lie awake at night and fail to get impressions out of his mind due to worry and anxiety. If he could forget them they would become beneficial agents working upon his ether body. This shows vividly that forgetting is a blessing, at the same time highlighting the importance of not compulsively clinging to some notion or other but instead learning to forget it. It is extremely injurious to a person's health if he cannot forget certain things.

These very mundane and momentary things also have their ethical and moral dimension. The character of someone who does not harbour grudges has a beneficial effect, and there is really a connection here. To harbour grudges eats away at a person's health. If someone has done harm to us and, having absorbed the impression of what he did to us we repeatedly return to it whenever we see him, then we relate this idea of harm to the person concerned, and allow it to stream out from us. But if the next time we see this person, we manage to shake his hand as if nothing has happened, this is actually healing—not just in a metaphorical sense but in reality. A notion that appears dull and ineffective outwardly when someone has injured us can at the same time pour into us and act in many ways as an inwardly healing balm. These things are realities, and can again show us the broader aspects of the blessing of forgetting. Forgetting is not a mere deficiency in us but is intrinsic to the most beneficial aspects of human life. If we only developed our memory, with everything retained there that makes an impression on us, our ether body would accumulate ever more of a burden, acquiring more and more content but at the same time growing increasingly withered. We owe our capacity for development to forgetting. But it is also true to say that no idea vanishes entirely from us—and we can best see this in the great memory tableau of our life that unfolds before us immediately after death. Here we see that no impression is ever entirely lost.

We have touched upon the blessing of forgetting in daily life, both in neutral and moral realms. Let us now consider how forgetting works in the greater scope of life between death and a new birth. What is the nature of kamaloca, that period of transition we pass through before our entry into devachan, the true world of spirit? Kamaloca exists because immediately after death we cannot forget the inclinations, desires and pleasures we entertained during our lifetime. At death we first depart from our physical body, and then behold the great memory tableau I have often described. After two, three or at most four days this ceases entirely, leaving a kind of extract of the ether body. While the real, full part of the ether body draws away and dissolves into the general, universal ether, a kind of essence remains, the ether body's framework or matrix, but now contracted. The astral body is the bearer of all instincts, drives, desires, passions, feelings, emotions and pleasures. Now in kamaloca the astral body would be unable to become aware of the torments of privation if it were not continually able to recall, through its ongoing connection with the residues of the ether body, what it has enjoyed and desired in life. The shedding of these habits is basically nothing other than a gradual forgetting of what chains us to the physical world. And so, when a person wishes to enter devachan, he must first learn to forget what chains him to the physical world. Here too therefore we see that we are tormented by retaining our memory of the physical world. Just as anxieties can become a torment when they refuse to be dislodged from our memory, inclinations and instincts that remain after death are likewise a torment; and this tormenting memory of our connection with life comes to expression in everything we have to undergo during our kamaloca period. The moment we have succeeded in forgetting all desires and wishes connected with the physical world— and only then—the achievements and fruits of our previous life appear in the way necessary for them to take effect in devachan. There they create and craft the shape of our forthcoming life.

Basically, in devachan we work at the new form we are to have when we return to earthly life. This work of preparing the subsequent pattern of our being produces the bliss we experience in passing through devachan. Having undergone kamaloca, we begin to prepare our future form. Life in devachan is always taken up with using the essence accorded us to elaborate the archetype of our subsequent form. We create this archetype by working the fruits of our past life into it. But we can only do this by forgetting what made kamaloca so difficult for us.

In speaking of suffering and privation in kamaloca, we see that this is due to our inability to forget certain connections with the physical world, and that this world still hovers before us like a memory. Once we have traversed 'Lethe's flood', the river of oblivion, and learned to forget, the achievements and experiences of our previous incarnation are used gradually to develop the archetype, the prototype of our subsequent life. And then suffering starts to be replaced by the sacred bliss of devachan. Just as we can be plagued in ordinary life, to the point of ill health, by anxieties and images that refuse to fade from our memory, and become a dry, withering obstacle inserted in our etheric body, so in our being after death we bear an obstacle that will go on causing us suffering and privation until, by forgetting, we have swept aside all connections with the physical world. And just as these forgotten notions can become a seed of recovery for us, so all experiences of our past life become a wellspring of joy in devachan once we have traversed the river of oblivion, and have forgotten all that binds us to life in the world of the senses.

And thus we see how these laws of forgetting and remembering hold true for life in its broadest scope.

You may ask how, after death, we can have any notions whatever of what happened in our previous life if we are obliged to forget this life. You might wonder whether 'forgetting' is a concept that can be entertained at all since the human soul has cast off its ether body and, after all, memory and forgetting are connected with this body. Naturally, memory and forgetting acquire a somewhat different form after death. A transformation occurs so that in place of ordinary recall we read in the akashic record. Whatever has happened in the world does not vanish but exists objectively. As memory of our connection with physical life fades during kamaloca, these same occurrences surface in a quite different way, becoming apparent to us in the akashic record. We then no longer need the connection with our life as produced by ordinary memory. All such questions can be resolved if we take the time to ponder them: they only gradually become clear since it is not possible to explain everything at once.

To know of these things also helps us understand much in daily life. A good deal of what belongs to the human ether body becomes apparent in the way the temperaments affect us. We have seen that the enduring disposition we refer to as 'temperament' also has its source in the etheric body. Consider a person of melancholic temperament who cannot get over certain ideas that he feels compelled to keep pondering—quite different from a person of sanguine or phlegmatic temperament whose ideas fade as fast as they arise. A melancholic temperament, in precisely the way we have been describing, can be injurious to health, whereas a sanguine temperament can be exceedingly conducive to health in some respects. Of course this should not be taken to mean that we ought to try to forget everything. But the healthy, beneficial aspect of a sanguine or phlegmatic temperament can be understood precisely in relation to these things, and likewise the unhealthy aspect of a melancholic temperament. We will still need to ask whether the phlegmatic temperament acts in the right way. A phlegmatic who absorbs inconsequential ideas will soon forget them, and this can only be healthy for him. But if these are the only notions he absorbs, this will not be good after all. Diverse things, you see, are all interrelated here.

So let us ask again: Is forgetting a defect of human nature or does it have a beneficial aspect after all? Spiritual-scientific insights enable us to answer this question. And strong moral impulses, we find, can also follow from such insights. If a person believes that it is—quite objectively—conducive to his health and well-being to be able to forget insults and injuries to which he has been exposed, a quite different impulse will guide him. But as long as he thinks this has no effect, no moralizing sermon will do any good at all. By knowing that he needs to forget, and that his well-being depends on it, he will open himself to this impulse in a quite different way. This doesn't have to be merely egoistic. We can look at it like this: If I am sick and ailing, if I ruin the inner state of my spirit, soul and body, I will be of no use to the world. The question of well-being can be considered from an entirely different point of view. A pronounced egotist will anyway gain little from such considerations. But for someone concerned with the good of humanity, who therefore wishes to help further this—and keeping in mind his own well-being as part and parcel of it—such considerations will enable him to draw moral conclusions too if he can reflect upon such things. And then, if spiritual science enters and acts upon our life, revealing to us the truth about certain spiritual states, it will, more than any other insight, provide us too with the most powerful ethical and moral impulses rather than moral commandments of a merely external nature. Insight into the *realities* of the spiritual world, such as spiritual science conveys, provides a strong impetus to enhance and improve human life, also in the realm of moral conduct.

LECTURE 8

BERLIN, 10 NOVEMBER 1908

THOSE of you who have been attending these branch lectures for several years may have noticed that their themes are not randomly chosen but follow a certain sequence and progression. Even within the space of a single winter the lectures always have a certain inner connection even if this isn't immediately outwardly apparent. It will therefore be very important to take account of the various courses held here alongside the branch evenings themselves. The aim of the former is to bring members who have joined later up to date, as it were, on the stage we have reached with these branch lectures. Someone who joins us here will meet many things in branch lectures that cannot be easily understood without further explanation. But here I must mention something else that should increasingly be borne in mind in the various branches of our German section. Since a certain consecutive thread runs through the lectures, I am obliged to shape each one in a way that will inform the whole series. In a single branch lecture for more advanced members, it is impossible, therefore, to couch things in a way that is easily accessible to someone who has only been present for a short while. Of course one could speak about the same theme in a more elementary way, but this would be inappropriate when seeking, as we do, to progressively develop our spiritual-scientific life in the branch meetings. This is connected in turn with the fact that we should increasingly refrain—all the more so the further we progress—from publishing or reporting on the lectures I give in branch meetings, or even sharing them between branch groups. This should really be avoided. You see, increasingly it really does matter a great deal whether a lecture given in a branch on a Monday is followed, the following Monday, by the next consecutive lecture. Even if members of the audience do not immediately see how the latter follows the former, it is important. By passing such lectures around, no account can be taken of the context involved. In some circumstances, a subsequent lecture is read before a previous one, inevitably leading to misunderstandings and confusion. I mention this as an important aspect of our anthroposophical life. Even a parenthesis, or greater or lesser accentuation of a word or phrase, is connected with the whole developing trajectory of our branch life. And only if publication of the lectures is strictly monitored so that, basically, nothing is published before I have checked it, can copying or publishing of lectures have a beneficial outcome.

In a sense this is also a kind of introduction to the forthcoming lectures to be given here in our branch. During the winter an inner thread will run through the sequence of lectures: the preparatory material will culminate, especially in this winter's lectures, in a quite specific, concluding focus. The lecture given here a week ago was a small beginning, and today's will be a kind of continuation—not, though, in the sense of fiction instalments in a magazine, in which the thirty-eighth instalment picks up where the thirty-seventh left off. Instead, everything will be *inwardly* interrelated, even if the topics appear to be different, and the connection will lie in an eventual culmination in the final lectures. Today, therefore, in relation to these final lectures, I will already offer some brief comments on the nature of illness; and next Monday I will speak about the origin, historical significance and meaning of the Ten Commandments. It might appear that there is no connection at all between these. You will find in the end, however, that there really is an inner connection between all these things, and that they are not presented as distinct and separate lectures—as might well be the case for a broader public.

Today we will discuss the nature of illness, of diseases, from the point of view of spiritual science. People usually only concern themselves with disease, or at least with one or other forms of disease, when they fall ill in some way; and then they are mostly only interested in their recovery, in the fact of being cured. *How* they are cured is usually of very little interest to them, and it is even very agreeable to them not to have to concern themselves further with the nature of this recovery. Most of our contemporaries are happy to delegate the task of curing them to the people appointed to do so. In fact, a far more pervasive faith in authority holds sway in this field in our era than has ever held sway in the sphere of religion. Medical papacy, irrespective of what form it assumes in one place or another, has today become extremely prevalent and will go on taking stronger hold in future. Lay people are not in the least at fault for this state of affairs and its future increase. You see, people don't give it any thought, don't concern themselves with such things—not, at least, until they have first-hand experience of it, suffer an acute illness and need a cure. And for this reason a great majority of the population looks on with complete indifference as the medical papacy assumes ever greater proportions, worming its way into the most diverse fields—for instance, intervening extensively in children's education, in school life, and staking a claim here to a certain form of therapy. People do not worry about the deeper underlying factors at work here. They stand by and watch as public ordinances are given some kind of legislative form. They have no real wish to gain insight into such things. By contrast there will always be those who, finding themselves in difficulty and discovering that ordinary, materialistic medicine—whose foundations they have no interest in—does not answer their needs, will seek help from practitioners who draw on an esoteric foundation. But still they will be concerned only with whether or not they can be cured. They are blithely unconcerned as to whether all mainstream methods and knowledge are undermining and undercutting a deeper, spiritually derived approach. Who worries if a public ordinance prohibits the practice of a method founded on esoteric insight, or even if the practitioner is locked up? People fail to consider all such things thoroughly enough, and only wake up to them in a particular case that affects them directly. The task of an authentic spiritual movement, though, is to waken awareness that the egotistic quest for a cure is insufficient, but that instead insight is needed into the deeper foundations of these things, and the dissemination of such insight.

In our materialistic age it is all too obvious to anyone who can see what is going on that medical ideas in particular are most powerfully influenced by the materialistic mode of thinking. But to chase after a catch-all phrase, lauding one method or another, and merely criticizing what is based on scientific foundations—and is, in many respects useful, but is nevertheless dressed up in materialistic theories—will be just as mistaken as, on the other hand, to subsume everything under 'psychic healing' and all such one-sided approaches. Above all, modern humanity must increasingly realize that the human being is a complex entity, and that everything relating to us is informed by such complexity. If a scientific discipline maintains that we consist only of the physical body, it will be unable to engage in any salutary way with aspects of human health or disease. You see, health and illness relate to the whole human being, and not just to the part of him that is the physical body.

But here again we should not regard the matter in too superficial a way. There are plenty of properly qualified physicians who certainly will not accept that their faith is rooted in materialism but instead will profess one religious faith or another. They would be indignant if you reproached them with having a deeply materialistic outlook. But this isn't what counts. What somebody says, and his convictions, have no significance at all—that's his personal affair. In actual practice what counts is that one can apply realities that are not just present in the sensory world but infuse and permeate the world of spirit, and can make practical use of them. However pious a doctor may be, and however many ideas he may have about some kind of world of spirit, if his medical practice is based on rules founded entirely on our materialistic world-view, and if he tries to cure, therefore, in a way that only acknowledges the body, he is still a materialist, however theoretically spiritual his outlook. What someone says or believes does not count compared to his ability to bring the powers underlying the visible sense world into living movement. It is likewise of little purpose to disseminate an anthroposophical doctrine of fourfold human nature, prattling on about physical body, ether body, astral body and I—even if we can in some way define and describe these things. That too is not the important thing. Instead we need to understand increasingly the living interplay of these levels of the human being: to understand how physical body, ether body, astral body and I are involved in human health and disease, and what acts in reciprocal connection with these aspects. For instance, if we never take account of what spiritual science can tell us about the nature of the fourth level of the human being, the I, however much anatomy and physiology we study we will never gain insight into the nature of the blood. It's simply impossible. And for this reason we will never in a million years be able to say anything significant or useful about diseases connected with the blood and its nature. The blood is the expression of our I nature. There is actually a great deal of truth in the old saying which Goethe includes in his *Faust*, that 'Blood is a very special fluid.'[19] Modern scientists have no inkling that their research should attend to our physical blood in a quite different way from other aspects of human physical corporeality—which are the expression of something quite different again. Our glands are the expression, the physical counterpart of the etheric body, and we have to regard what constitutes such a gland, whether liver or pancreas, say, as something quite different from what we find in the blood as the expression of a much higher level of the human being—the I. And research methods must take due account of this, showing us how we should approach these things. Now, though, I wish to say something that will really only be comprehensible to an advanced student of anthroposophy, but which it is still important to state.

To materialistically minded academics of today it seems quite evident that if one makes an incision in the body, the blood that flows from this can be studied by all the available means. So they describe it: this is blood—roughly as one would describe any other substance, an acid or suchlike, according to chemical research methods that govern modern procedures. But in doing so they overlook something that is, in fact, not only unknown to materialistic science but must seem to be idiocy and fantasy, yet is nevertheless true: the blood running in your veins that sustains the living body is not at all what flows out when I make an incision and produce a red drop. The moment blood leaves the body, it undergoes a transformation that renders it quite different. What flows out as congealing blood, however fresh it may be, is not indicative of the whole essence within the living organism. Blood is the expression of the I, a high aspect of the human being. Even in physical terms, blood is something whose totality you simply cannot study physically—because, when you see it, it is no longer at all the same as it was when flowing in the body. It cannot be physically observed, for the moment it is brought to view to be studied by some method like X-ray examination, it is no longer the blood itself at all that is being studied but instead just the external reflection of blood in the physical domain. People will only gradually come to understand these things. There have always been researchers who drew on esoteric foundations and said this, but they have been dismissed as fantasists, philosophers or suchlike.

In states of human health or disease everything is really connected with our fourfold human nature, with our full complexity. This is why we can only understand a healthy or sick person by drawing on spiritual-scientific insight into the human being. There are quite specific types of debility in the human constitution that can only be understood when we realize they are connected with the nature of the I, and that in a sense—though within certain limits—they are in turn revealed in the blood as expression of the I. Then there are certain types of debility in the human organism that can be attributed to a malfunction of the astral body, thus affecting the astral body's outward expression, the nervous system. But in this second instance you will have to take note of the subtlety needed to approach such things. When the human astral body bears within it the kind of irregularity that comes to expression in the nervous system as the outward reflection of the astral body, we initially find that the nervous system shows a certain physical, functional incapacity. If the nervous system cannot function properly in a certain direction, this incapacity can result in all sorts of symptoms affecting the stomach, head and heart. Yet a disorder whose symptoms become apparent in the stomach cannot necessarily be attributed to a certain type of nervous system malfunction, and thus to its source in the astral body; it may have an entirely different cause.

The types of disease that are connected with the I itself and thus with its outward expression, the blood, usually manifest as chronic diseases—but only *usually*, since in reality things are not so neatly compartmentalized, although sharp demarcations can be drawn when making observations. What can generally first be observed as a particular debility is usually a symptom. Some symptom or other can appear, but there is an underlying debility of the blood, and this has its origin in an irregularity of the aspect of the human being we call the I-bearer. I could speak to you for hours about types of chronic disease which originate in the blood, in physical terms, and in the I in spiritual terms. These are primarily genetic diseases in the true sense, passing from one generation to the next. And it is these diseases that can only be understood if we consider human nature from a spiritual point of view.

Let's take a patient who has a chronic condition—which basically means that he is never really well. He suffers sometimes from one thing, sometimes from another, from one illness or another. Here we have to take a deeper look at the underlying cause, and above all be able to take note of the real, fundamental character of the I. What kind of person is this really? If we know something in this field that fully accords with life itself, we can see that quite specific types of chronic disease are connected with a particular underlying, purely soul-related character of the I. Certain chronic diseases will never appear in someone whose character is informed by gravity and dignity, but they will in a person disposed to whistle and sing. I can only mention these things in passing here, as a waymarker in these preparatory lectures.

But you see, if someone comes along who says, 'I've had a certain condition for years now,' it is important to be generally clear first of all what kind of person this is. We have to know the underlying character and nuance of his I, otherwise we will inevitably get the symptoms wrong unless guided by very lucky chance. The important thing in relation to curing these diseases which are, at the same time, genetic or hereditary in the truest sense, is to take account of the person's whole surroundings in so far as they can exert a direct or indirect influence on his I. Once we have really got to know someone in this way, we may sometimes judge it advisable to send him, if possible, to a particular kind of natural environment during the winter. Or we may recommend that he change his profession if he has a particular kind of job, and instead explore a different aspect of life. Here it will chiefly be important to adopt measures that can exert the right influence on the character of the I. Someone who wishes to cure patients must have broad life experience so that he can enter into another's nature and recommend such things as a change of profession in order to effect a cure. The emphasis must be on what a person's nature requires. In this domain in particular any chance of a cure may perhaps fail sometimes because such measures cannot be carried out. But in many cases such measures can be adopted once we know what they are. A great deal can be achieved for some people for instance if they live in a mountainous region rather than at sea level. These are things relating to diseases that outwardly manifest as chronic diseases and are physically connected with the blood, and spiritually with the nature of the I.

We now come to diseases which—in spiritual terms—are primarily rooted in irregularities of the astral body, and manifest in certain incapacities of the nervous system in one or another direction. A great many—or even most—common acute diseases are connected with what we have referred to above. You see, it is misguided to think, as people often do, that a stomach or heart condition, or even some clearly perceptible irregularity somewhere, can be fully cured by working on these symptoms directly. The major aspect of this symptom may be that the nervous system is incapable of functioning properly here. Thus a heart disorder may simply be due to an associated malfunction of the nervous system, and therefore a failure to support the heart's movements. Here it is quite unnecessary to maltreat the heart—or in another instance the stomach—for basically nothing is directly wrong with them; it is just that the nerves that should be supporting the organ are incapable of functioning properly. If someone has this type of stomach disorder and we administer betaine hydrochloride, this would be the same kind of mistake as imagining that because a train arrives late there is something wrong with the locomotive itself, and starting to tinker with it. It will still arrive late because the cause, if one looks, turns out to be the train driver getting drunk each time he's meant to drive the engine. The right thing to do, therefore, would be to start with the train driver, who, after all, is the cause of the late arrival of the train. In the same way, in stomach complaints, we may have to address the nerves that look after the stomach instead of starting with the stomach itself. In materialistic medicine, too, you may find some such remarks. But we are not saying that a stomach disorder should always direct you to look first at the nerves taking care of it, for that again will achieve nothing. We will only get somewhere if we know that the nerve is an expression of the astral body, and that we can trace things back to the constitution of the astral body and seek the causes of a complaint in its irregularities. Then the question arises as to how we can proceed.

In treating disorders of this nature, initially we will need to adopt a dietary cure, using the right combination of foods and what the person in question relishes. Thus we focus on his mode of life, not as concerns outward things but in relation to what he digests and assimilates. And this is something into which no insight can ever be gained through a merely materialistic science. Here we must realize that everything surrounding us in the macrocosm of the wider world is related to our complex internal organism, to the microcosm. Every food we know, therefore, is connected in a quite specific way to what lies within us. We have spent much time acquainting ourselves with the long progress of human evolution, and with discovering how all external nature has been formed by being ejected from the human being. In diverse studies we have repeatedly returned to the time of ancient Saturn, finding that nothing existed there apart from the human being himself, and that in a sense the human being, human evolution, secreted the other kingdoms of nature—the plant and animal realms and so forth. In the course of this evolution the formation of our organs corresponded entirely with what they expelled. As the mineral realm was expelled, quite specific internal organs arose. The heart could not have formed if certain plants, minerals and mineral capacities had not developed outwardly over the course of time. What developed in the external world has a particular relationship with what formed within us. And now anyone who knows how outer things relate to internal ones can say in each instance how an external substance in the macrocosm can be used to benefit the microcosm. Otherwise we can experience, in a sense, how what we stuff ourselves with really isn't suitable for us. We must therefore seek in spiritual science for the real foundations governing our judgement. When someone falls ill and his diet is then guided by purely empirical laws derived from statistics or chemistry, this will always be a superficial approach. We need a quite different rationale. Here, therefore, we see how spiritual insight has to stream and shine through everything connected with human health and disease.

Then there are certain diseases which can assume either more chronic or more acute forms, but which are connected with the human ether body, and therefore manifest in human glands. These diseases usually have nothing at all to do with hereditary transmission, but instead are very much connected with a particular nation, race or people. In relation to diseases rooted in the ether body, therefore, which manifest as glandular diseases, we must always consider whether the patient is, say, Russian, Italian, Norwegian or French. These diseases are connected with national character and therefore manifest in very different ways. In the medical field, the following major error is made, for instance. Throughout Europe a very erroneous view of tabes or locomotor ataxia has become established. While it is assessed correctly for the population of western Europe, this is quite wrong as far as eastern Europeans are concerned, since it has a different origin there. Today these things vary very greatly. So now you will understand that this requires fairly careful attention as regards the particular mix of a population. We can only form any kind of judgement here if we learn to make distinctions about inner human nature. Today these diseases are treated in a merely external way, lumped together with the acute diseases, whereas in reality they belong to a quite different domain.

We must be aware of one thing especially: that those human organs which are subject to the influence of the ether body, and which can become diseased due to irregularities of the ether body, have very specific reciprocal relationships. Thus for instance there is a very specific relationship between a person's brain and heart; and we can express this in a more pictorial way by saying that this mutual relationship between brain and heart corresponds to the relationship between sun and moon—with the heart corresponding to the sun here, and the brain to the moon. And so here we must be clear that if, say, a disease of the heart arises it will—in so far as it is rooted in the etheric body—inevitably work back upon the brain, just as a solar phenomenon such as an eclipse must affect the moon. It really amounts to the same thing since there is a direct connection here.

In esoteric medicine these connections are also indicated by using the heavenly bodies as pictures relating to the constellation of diverse human organs: the heart as sun, brain as moon, spleen as Saturn, liver as Jupiter, gall bladder as Mars, kidneys as Venus and lungs as Mercury. If you study the mutual relationships of the constellations you gain a picture of the mutual relationships between human organs in so far as these involve the ether body. It is impossible for the gall bladder to become diseased—a condition which must therefore be traced spiritually to the ether body—without this having concomitant effects of some kind on the organs named above. If we see the gall bladder in terms of Mars, then it acts in the same way as Mars does within our planetary system. In the case of a disease involving the etheric body we have to know how the organs are interrelated; and yet such diseases are primarily those which we should treat with specific medicines—and this shows us that we should avoid all one-sided views in the esoteric domain. Here we resort to medicines that are found in the external world in plants and minerals. The properties of plants and minerals have great significance for the nature of the etheric body. So if we know that a disease originates in the etheric body, and therefore manifests in the glandular system in a certain way, we must find medicines that properly redress or repair the complex of interactions. Specifically targeted medicines can be used primarily in diseases of this kind, where the prime factor is, of course, their origin in the ether body, followed by their connection with national character and the fact that the organs interact in such conditions.

But you may now have gained the idea that if we cannot relocate someone because of his professional ties or for some other reason, then we will be unable to help him. But there is another effective approach, which draws on the human psyche. This 'psychological' method is most effective if the disease is to be sought in a person's actual ego or I. If a chronic disease of this kind arises, in some way rooted in the blood, the psychological remedies come into their own. If carried out in the right way, their action upon the I can fully replace external influences streaming into us. Here you will be able to discern everywhere a subtle, intimate connection if you observe what the human soul can experience if, say, a person has had his nose to the grindstone and then briefly enjoys some country air. The feelings of joy that lift the soul are something we can call a 'psychological' method in the broadest sense. But if a physician practises the right methodology, his personal influence can gradually replace this. Psychological methods are most justified in such conditions. We cannot ignore them if only because most illnesses originate in an irregularity of the human I.

We now come to the diseases that arise due to irregularities of the astral body. Here, although we can still use solely psychological methods, they have much less value and will therefore be used less often in treatment. Instead we use dietetic healing methods. Only in the third type of diseases, as we have called them, is it really justified to support the healing process with external medicines. If we observe the complexity of the human being, healing too must be seen in a holistic and not a one-sided way.

The last category of diseases are 'diseases proper'—those that originate in and relate to the physical body. These are the true infectious diseases. This is an important subject, which we will return to in more detail in one of the subsequent lectures after considering the true origin of the 'Ten Commandments'. As you will see, these things are certainly connected. Today I can only indicate that this fourth type of disease exists, and that in discerning its deep foundations we require knowledge of the whole of nature, with which the human physical body is connected. The physical is not what underlies this, but really once more, and even more so, the realm of spirit. Even having considered this form of illness, we will not yet have exhausted all major types of disease; we will see that human karma also plays into it as a fifth aspect that we have to include.

Gradually therefore we will see how the five different forms of human disease reveal something of their nature as disorders originating in the domain of the I, astral body, etheric body, physical body, and what we can regard as karmically determined aspects of disease. The whole modern medical outlook will only lead to something salutary when it is imbued with insight into the higher aspects of human nature. Until then we will not have a school of medicine that can really engage with what is needed. Although these things, like many of our esoteric insights, must be brought into a form appropriate for the modern world, you should remember that they are, in a sense, an ancient form of wisdom.

Medicine was originally based on spiritual perception and gradually became ever more materialistic. More than in any other field of knowledge, perhaps, medicine can show us how materialism has taken humanity by storm. In former times, at least, people were aware that knowledge of fourfold human nature was needed to understand the human being. Naturally materialism had earlier forerunners, so that even four hundred years ago and more, clairvoyant people could see that everyone around them was starting to think in a materialistic way. Paracelsus,[20] for example, who is not understood today but regarded as a fantasist or dreamer, asserted in no uncertain terms that medical science of his day, as propounded in Salerno, Montpellier or Paris, and also in areas of Germany, was materialistic, or at least was on the way to becoming so. Because of his world standing, Paracelsus saw the need— as is again necessary today—to draw attention to the nature of a medical outlook founded on the spirit as opposed to one acquired in a merely materialistic domain. Today it may be even more difficult than Paracelsus found, in his day, to make any headway with a Paracelsian mode of thinking. At that time medicine's materialistic outlook was not yet so sharply antagonistic to the thinking of Paracelsus as materialistic science is today to insight of any kind into the fundamentally spiritual nature of the human being. What Paracelsus said in relation to this still holds true today, therefore, but its validity is perceived still less. If you look at the thinking of people today who work at the dissection table or in the laboratory, and see how modern research is used to understand health and sickness, it would be very easy to oppose this materialistic outlook in the same way that Paracelsus did. The difference is that, unlike Paracelsus, one can have little hope that one might be understood or at least perhaps forgiven by contemporary physicians—*forgiven*, since Paracelsus himself stated that he had never rubbed shoulders with the upper classes, that he was not a refined fellow but came from a rough, working background and had grown up in a world of cheese, milk and oatbread, and therefore asked to be pardoned if what he said was not always couched in elegant language.

In discussing various dispositions to illness, Paracelsus says of both French, Italian and also German physicians:

> For it is a great error and much amiss that so many French and
> Italian physicians, especially in Montpellier, Salerno and Paris,

who wish to be lauded above all others and who despise everyone else, in fact know nothing themselves and have no skill but, as can be shown, their art is nothing but talk and pomp and much prattling. They are not ashamed to use clysters and purges, or bleed someone to death if it accords with their notions. They pride themselves on their knowledge and use of anatomy, but have never yet noticed that tartar accumulates in the teeth, not to mention all sorts of other conditions. These eye doctors can't see what's right in front of their nose. What is all your skill and anatomy? It's as much use as codswallop, and your eyes are too few to see what's staring you in the face. The German cuckoo doctors are no better—thieves and young idiots who, when they've seen everything know less than before. So they're drowning in muck and cadavers, and then it's funeral time for poor wash-rags—folk remedies would serve them much better![21]

LECTURE 9

BERLIN, 16 NOVEMBER 1908

CONTINUING from the start we made a week ago when we considered different forms of illness and human health, over the course of this winter we will look in ever greater detail at related matters. All our observations will culminate in a more precise understanding of human nature in general than we have gained so far through anthroposophy. Today's observations, as part of the overall sequence, will address the nature and significance of the Ten Commandments of Moses, since we will need to return to this later. First, we will discuss the profound significance of terms such as original sin and redemption, and will find that these concepts can regain their meaning in the light of what we have accomplished most recently, also in the field of science. To do so, however, we first need to examine the fundamental nature of the remarkable document that has come down to us from ancient days of Hebrew history, and appears to us as one of the most important building stones of the temple established as a kind of antechamber to Christianity. Such a document, particularly, can show us how little the form of the Bible we know today accords with it. The details I presented in the last two public lectures on 'The Bible and Wisdom'[22] will have given you the sense that it would be wrong to think that I was just citing certain [passages taken from] the translations and that such precise details are of no real importance. To think like this would be very superficial. Just recall for a moment that, as I pointed out,[23] a correct translation of verse 4 of the second chapter of Genesis ought to be, 'What follows here will tell of the generations, or of what issues from heaven and earth',[24] and that in Genesis the same word is used here for 'the descendants of heaven and earth' as later, in the passage 'This is the book about the generations—or the descendants—of Adam.'[25] In both cases the same word is used. And there is great significance in the fact that, where the human being is described as coming forth from heaven and earth, the same word is used as later when speaking of the generations descended from Adam. Such things are not just some kind of pedantic amendment that slightly improves the translation, but they go to the very heart not only of our translation but of our understanding of this ancient document of humanity. We actually draw on the well-springs of our anthroposophical world-view, you can say, in regarding one of the most important tasks of this world-view, of anthroposophy itself, as being to give back the Bible to humanity in a true form. Here we are primarily interested in what has been said in general about the Ten Commandments.

These Ten Commandments are regarded today by most people as laws decreed in the same way that some modern government might enshrine them. It will be admitted, of course, that these laws contained in the Ten Commandments are more comprehensive and more general, and hold good beyond their particular time and locality. Yet although regarded as more general laws, people will think that really they just have the same effect or goal as modern legislation. In fact this overlooks the real lifeblood that pulses in these Ten Commandments. We can tell that this has been misperceived because all the translations accessible to us today have unwittingly incorporated a really very superficial explanation that does not accord at all with the spirit of these Ten Commandments. If we engage with this spirit, you will see how the meaning of the Ten Commandments is integrated into observations we have embarked on—although it may appear as if we are taking an irrelevant sideways leap here in considering them.

Above all, as a kind of introduction, allow me to attempt to offer a somewhat fitting German version of the Ten Commandments, and only then proceed further. This 'translation', if one can call it that, will require some further honing. But the lifeblood, the real meaning, will first be conveyed with this German version, as we will see directly. If we translate the sense of the Ten Commandments—not translating word for word with a dictionary in hand, which will lead to the worst possible outcome since what counts is the essence of the words, the whole soul significance they had for their time—we get the following:

> First commandment: I am the eternal divine that you sense within you. I led you out of the land of Egypt, where you could not hearken to Me in you. Henceforth, you shall not place other gods above Me. You shall not accept as higher gods whatever— working out of the earth or between heaven and earth—shows you an image of something that shines above in heaven. You shall not worship what, of all this, is lower than the divine in you. For I am the eternal in you, that works into the body and therefore works upon coming generations. I am divine nature whose influence persists. If you do not recognize Me in you, I will vanish as your divine nature in your children, grandchildren and great-grand-children, and their body will grow barren. If you recognize Me in you, I will live on as You through to the thousandth generation, and the bodies of your people will flourish.

> Second commandment: You shall not speak of Me in you in error, for every error regarding the I in you will corrupt your body.

> Third commandment: You shall divide working day from feast day, so that your existence becomes an image of My existence. For what lives in you as I, made the world in six days, and on the seventh day lived within itself. Therefore your actions and those of your sons and your daughters, and your servants' actions, and those of your cattle, and of all else that dwells with you, shall be directed outwardly for only six days; but on the seventh day your gaze shall seek Me.

> Fourth commandment: Uphold the ways of your father and mother, so that you shall remain in possession of the estate that they have acquired through the power I have developed in them.

> Fifth commandment: You shall not commit murder.

> Sixth commandment: You shall not break wedlock.

Seventh commandment: You shall not steal.

Eighth commandment: You shall not belittle the worth of your neighbour by speaking untruth of him.

Ninth commandment: You shall not look enviously upon the property your neighbour owns.

Tenth commandment: You shall not look enviously upon your neighbour's wife nor upon the helpmates and other beings through whom he finds his further advancement.

Let us ask what these Ten Commandments chiefly tell us. We will see that both in the latter part, where this is less apparent, as well as the first part, the Jewish people are told through Moses that the power that proclaimed itself to Moses in the burning thorn bush with words designating its name, 'I am the I am'—'Ehyeh asher ehyeh!'[26]—is henceforth to dwell with them. I have mentioned that other peoples at that point in evolution were not able to recognize the 'I am', the original ground of the fourth aspect of the human being, so clearly or vividly as was intended for the Jewish people. The God who poured a drop of his being into human beings, so enabling the fourth aspect of the human entelechy to become the bearer of this drop, the I-bearer, comes to his people's awareness through Moses. We can therefore say that the Ten Commandments are founded on the view that Yahweh-God laboured and worked to further humanity's upward evolution, to reach this point too. Yet it is also true that the work of spiritual entities is already underway before their influence is clearly perceived. What worked in ancient peoples of pre-Mosaic times took effect in them, it is true, but it was only proclaimed as a concept and idea, as an active power within the human soul, by Moses to his people. The whole, encompassing effect of feeling oneself to be an I to the degree experienced by the Jewish people, was made clear to them, and this was the important thing. In this people we must regard the Yahweh being as a kind of transitional being: Yahweh is the being who pours the divine drop into each person's own human individuality. Yet he is, at the same time, a God of the whole race. The individual Jew still felt himself, in a sense, to be united with the I that also lived in Abraham's incarnation, and streamed down through the whole Jewish people. The Jewish people felt connected with the God of Abraham, Isaac and Jacob.[27] It was an era of transition, and things would only change radically when Christianity was proclaimed. But what was to come to earth through Christ is proclaimed in advance in the Old Testament, above all through what Moses tells his people. Thus we see the full power of I-realization pour gradually into the Jewish people during the course of history described in the Old Testament. The Jewish people were intended to become fully aware of the effect on a person's whole life of no longer living in a kind of unconscious state about the I, but instead learning to feel within himself the I, the 'I am the I am'[28] as the name of God, in its full effect on the inmost soul.

Today people have only an abstract sense of these things. If we speak of the I today, and what is connected with it, they hear it as mere words. At the time when this I was first proclaimed to the Jewish people in the figure of the ancient Yahweh-God, they felt this I as the influx of a power that enters the human being and changes the whole configuration of his astral body, etheric body and physical body. And this people had to be told that the conditions governing their life and health were different when the I did not yet live in their soul as awareness; that health and sickness had previously been governed by different conditions than they were now becoming, and that this change would affect their whole lives. It was therefore important to describe to the Jewish people the new conditions they were entering into: that they should no longer merely look upwards to heaven or downwards to the earth when speaking of gods, but should gaze into their own soul. Looking inwards into the soul in a truthful way invokes right living, and works all the way through into health. This awareness certainly underlies the Ten Commandments, whereas a false view of what entered the soul as the I withers a person and destroys him. We need really only study historical documents to discover how little these Ten Commandments were intended as merely external laws, but instead were thought of in the way I have described: as something of the most incisive importance for the health and wholesomeness of astral, etheric and physical body. But who reads books today with care and accuracy? One need only read on a few pages [in the Bible] to find, in a further elaboration of the Ten

Commandments, that the Jewish people were told of their effects on the whole human being. There it is stated: 'I will take sickness away from the midst of thee. There shall nothing cast their young, nor be barren, in thy land: the number of thy days I will fulfil.'[29]

This means: When the I comes to expression in a way that is permeated by the nature of the Ten Commandments, one of the results will be that you cannot fall sick and die in the flower of your years, but that, through the properly grasped I, something will be able to stream into the three bodies—astral body, ether body and physical body—which will allow you to reach the full tally of your years, so that you stay healthy into ripe old age. This is clearly stated. But it is necessary to delve deeply into these things. Modern theologians, however, do not find this so easy. A popular little pamphlet[30]—whose cover price of a few pennies already arouses one's irritation—says the following of the Ten Commandments: that it is easy to find in them the chief laws governing human life; in one half the laws relating to our conduct towards God and in the other half those relating to our conduct towards human beings. To make things clear and understandable, the author says that the fourth commandment should be included in the first half relating to God. The fact that this gentleman manages to make one 'half' of four and the other of six is just a small indication of how people tackle things today. The rest of the book goes on in the same kind of vein—as if four were the same as six.

We are concerned here with the explanation given to the Jewish people of the right way for the I to permeate the three human levels or aspects. The most important thing—which we meet already in the first commandment—is the statement: If you become aware of this I as a spark of divinity, you must experience in the I a spark, an emanation of the highest, most powerful divinity which participates in the creation of the earth.

Let us remind ourselves what we have learned about the human being's evolution. We said that the human physical body arose during existence on ancient or old Saturn, where gods were working upon it. Then, on old Sun, the ether body was added. The way in which both bodies were further elaborated was likewise the work of divine, spiritual beings. Then, on old Moon, the astral body was incorporated—all as the work of divine, spiritual beings. What then made us into human beings in the sense we understand it today was the incorporation of our I on earth. The highest divine power collaborated in this. Therefore, as long as the human being was not yet able to become fully conscious of this fourth aspect, he could not have any intimation, either, of the highest divine power that participates in his development and exists within him. As a human being we have to say that divine beings worked upon my physical body, but these are not as great as the Godhead that has now endowed me with the I. The same is true of ether body and astral body. The Jewish people therefore, who first received the prophetic annunciation of this I, had to be made aware that the peoples around them worshipped gods who, in accordance with their current stage of evolution, can work upon astral body, ether body and physical body. But they cannot work upon the I. This God, who works in the I, was always present. He announced himself in his creative workings. But only now did he proclaim his name.

In recognizing and paying tribute to the other gods, the human being is not free. Here he is a being who worships the gods of his lower aspects. But when the human being becomes aware of the God of whom a part exists in his I, then he is a free being—one who relates to his fellow men as a free being. Today we do not have the same relationship to our astral body, ether body and physical body as we do to our I. We inhabit this I, as the entity with which we are in closest direct connection. We will only have such a relationship to our astral body once we have transformed it into Manas; and to our ether body when we have transformed it into Buddhi, developing it into divine nature through our I. Although the I was the last aspect to emerge, it is nevertheless the one in which we dwell. And when we encompass the I, we therefore encompass something in which the divine comes to meet us in its immediate, most intrinsic form. The current forms of our astral body, ether body and physical body, by contrast, were configured by preceding gods. Thus unlike the people of Israel, other peoples around them worshipped divinities who had worked upon these lower aspects of the human being. And when an image was made of these lower divinities, it resembled some form or other that existed on earth or in the sky, or between the sky and earth. For, you see, all we bear within us is spread out through the rest of nature. If we make images of the mineral realm they can only represent to us the gods who worked on the physical body. If we make images out of the plant kingdom, they can only represent to us the divinities who worked on the ether body, since we have the ether body in common with the world of plants. And images drawn from the animal kingdom can only symbolize for us the gods who worked on the astral body. But what makes the human being the crowning glory of Creation is what he encompasses in his I. No outer image can express this. And this was why it had to be explained and emphasized to the Jewish people, in no uncertain terms, that they contained within them a direct emanation of the current highest level of divine nature, which could not be symbolized in an image drawn from the mineral, plant or animal kingdom, however lofty such an image might be. All gods worshipped in this way, they were told, are lower than the God who lives in their I. If they desired to worship *this* God within them, the others must withdraw—and then the Jewish people would bear within them the healthy, true power of their I.

What we find straight away in the first of the Ten Commandments is therefore connected with the deepest mysteries of human evolution: 'I am the eternal divine nature that you sense within you. The power that I planted in your I became the impetus, the strength to lead you out of the land of Egypt, where you were unable to follow or hearken to Me within you.'

Moses led his people out of Egypt. And to make all this quite clear to us, special emphasis is placed on the fact that Yahweh wished to make his people into a nation of priests. The wise priests of other nations were those who were free as distinct from the rest of the people. Such emancipated figures knew of the great secret of the I, and also of the I-God who could not be pictorially represented. In such lands therefore there was a division between the wise priests, aware of the I, and the great, unliberated masses who could only hear and obey what the priests, in their strictest authority, permitted to issue from the mysteries. Individual members of the people did not have this immediate relationship, but instead the wise priests mediated it to them, and therefore all well-being and wholesomeness in life depended on the former. Well-being and health depended on the way they established institutions and organized everything. I would have to speak at great length to describe the deeper meaning of the Egyptian temple sleep to you and its effect on the nation's health; to describe the healing folk remedies that emanated from such rites—such as the Apis culture. Amongst a people of this kind, the whole nation was governed and guided through initiate leadership that enabled healing fluidae to emanate from these mystery centres. This was now set to change. The Jewish people were to become a nation of priests. Every single individual was to feel within himself a spark of this Yahweh God, and enter into a direct relationship with him. No longer was the wise figure of the priest to act as sole mediator. And therefore the whole people had to be instructed in this, being shown that false images—thus the lower images of the highest God—also have an unsalutory effect. This brings us to a domain which it is hard for modern people to gain any idea about, resulting in enormous transgressions.

Only if we can delve into spiritual science can we discover the mysterious way in which health and sickness develop. If you walk through the streets of a city, the atrocious things in advertisements and shop windows exert a baleful influence on your soul. Materialistic scientists have no sense at all of the capacity of these dire things to cause disease. They seek pathogens merely in bacilli, unaware that health and sickness are introduced into the body via the soul. Here only a humanity that acquaints itself with spiritual science will learn the significance of absorbing one or another kind of pictorial image.

Above all, the first commandment states that henceforth a person must be able to conceive how, above and beyond what is expressed in pictorial images, a non-pictorial impulse borders on the supersensible realm at this 'I point'. 'Strongly feel this I within you, and feel it such that a divine nature, higher than anything you can express in an image, weaves and surges through you in this I. In such a feeling you have a salutary power that will render you healthy in physical, ether and astral body!' A strong, health-giving I impulse was to be mediated here to the Jewish people. If this I is rightly recognized, then astral, etheric and physical bodies will be well formed, thus engendering strong life forces and health-bestowing powers which, emanating from each individual, are conveyed to the whole people. Since the tradition was to think of a people in terms of a thousand generations, the Yahweh God stated that proper incorporation of the I would render the human being a source of radiating health, and the people, as the Bible expresses it, would remain a healthy nation 'through to the thousandth generation'. But if the I is not understood in the right way, the body withers and becomes sick and ailing. If a father does not properly integrate the nature of the I in his soul, his body will become sick and ailing and the I will gradually withdraw; his son will be still more ailing, the grandson even more so; and ultimately we will be left only with an empty casing from which the Yahweh God has withdrawn. If the I impulse is not brought to bear, this lack will eventually work right through into the fourth aspect of our being and cause degeneration of the physical body.

Thus we see how, in the first of the Ten Commandments. Moses presents to the Jewish people the doctrine of the right action of the I:

> I am the eternal divine that you sense within you. I led you out of the land of Egypt, where you could not hearken to Me in you. Henceforth, you shall not place other gods above Me. You shall not accept as higher gods whatever, working out of the earth or between heaven and earth, shows you an image of something that shines above in heaven. You shall not worship what, of all this, is lower than the divine in you. For I am the eternal in you, that works into the body and therefore works upon coming generations. I am divine nature whose influence persists. If you do not recognize Me in you, I will vanish as your divine nature in your children, grandchildren and great-grandchildren, and their body will grow barren. If you recognize Me in you, I will live on as You into the thousandth generation, and the bodies of your people will flourish.

We can see here that this is not merely an abstract idea but something that should live and work right into the health of a people. The external process of health is led back to its origin in the spirit, which is proclaimed to humanity by developing degrees. The second commandment indicates this especially, where it is expressly said: 'You shall not form wrong ideas of my name, of what lives in you as I; for a true idea makes you healthy and full of life, and is wholesome for you, whereas a false idea will corrupt your body!' Thus every member of the Hebrew people of Moses is told, in particular, that whenever the name of God is uttered he should receive it as an admonishment to recognize the name of what has entered into him, as it lives within him, for this will engender health: 'You shall not speak of Me in you in error, for every error regarding the I in you will corrupt your body!'

And then, in the third commandment, we find a strict indication of the fact that, as an active, creating I, the human being is a microcosm. The Yahweh God created for six days and rested on the seventh, and this serves as an archetype to be reflected in human creativity. The third commandment expressly states: As a true I, you as a human being are also a reflection of your highest God, and in your deeds you should act as does your God! Thus human beings are urged here to ever more closely resemble the God who revealed himself to Moses in the burning bush:

> You shall divide working day from feast day, so that your existence may become an image of My existence. For what lives in you as I, made the world in six days, and on the seventh day lived within itself. Therefore your actions and those of your son and your daughter, and your servants' actions, and those of your cattle, and of all else that dwells with you, shall be directed outwardly for only six days; but on the seventh day your gaze shall seek Me in you.

Now the Ten Commandments start to increasingly focus on the individual. But this is always in the context of the idea of Yahweh or Jehovah being always at work as enduring power. In the fourth commandment we are led outwards from relationship with the supersensible to external sensory reality. This fourth commandment accentuates something very important, and this should be understood. Where a person enters existence as a self-aware I, he requires external means to enact this existence. He develops what we can call individual property and possessions. If we go back to the ancient Egyptian era, the great mass of the people do not yet have individual possessions in this way. We would find that only the wise priests make decisions about property. But now, with every individual seeking to develop an individual I, each person finds it necessary to intervene in external reality and have something of his own around him in order to embody his I in the outer world. The fourth commandment therefore indicates that a person who allows the individual I to work within him, acquires possessions, but that this property remains bound to the power of the I that endures in the Jewish people and is to be transmitted from father to son to grandson; and that the property the father owned will not be subject to the strong power of the I if the son should not continue the work of his father, under the sway of the father. It is therefore said: Let the I grow so strong in you that it endures and that, with the means the son inherits from the father, he may also preserve the means to live his way outwardly into his external surroundings.

Thus the conservatism of the spirit of ownership is intentionally given to the people of Moses at this period. The other laws, likewise, are underpinned by an awareness that occult forces underlie everything that happens in the world. Whereas today people regard the law of inheritance in only very external and abstract ways, those who properly understood the fourth commandment knew that spiritual powers are transmitted with inherited property, living on from one generation to the next, and intensifying I power. In this way the I power of each individual is enhanced by something that flows to it from the father's I power. The fourth commandment cannot be translated in a more grotesquely erroneous way than it usually is, for the real meaning is as follows: Strong I power should be developed in you, living on after you, and this shall pass to the son so that his I power shall be enhanced by something that can work on in him as the estate of his forefathers.

'Uphold the ways of your father and mother, so that you shall remain in possession of the estate that they have acquired through the power I have developed in them.'

And then all subsequent laws are also founded on the fact that human I power is enhanced through the proper realization of the I impulse, but that false employment of this will destroy it. The fifth commandment says something that can really only be properly understood through spiritual science. Everything connected with killing and destroying another's life weakens self-aware I power in the human being. By this means one can intensify black magic forces in a person, but only by enhancing human astral forces and bypassing I power.

Every form of killing destroys the divine nature of the perpetrator. This law does not therefore invoke something abstract but also something that allows esoteric forces to stream towards a person's I power when he enhances life, helps it to thrive and flourish, and does not destroy it. This is established here as an ideal for enhancement of individual I power; and only in less strongly accentuated domains is the same thing invoked in the sixth and seventh commandment.

Marriage establishes a centre for I power. Whoever breaks a marriage is therefore weakened in what should flow into I power. In the same way, anyone who desires to acquire possessions by taking or stealing from another, thus trying to deprive him of some of his I power, weakens his own I power. The guiding thought underlying this, too, is that the I should not weaken itself. And then, in the last three commandments, it is even indicated that giving a false direction to one's desires will also weaken I power. The life of desires has great significance for I power. Love enhances the power of the I while resentment or hatred lays waste to it. If a person hates another, therefore, disparaging him by saying something untrue about him, he weakens I power, diminishing the health and life force of everything around him. The same is true of envy of another's possessions. Merely desiring another's possessions renders his I power weak. The same is said in the tenth commandment of someone who looks enviously on the way in which his neighbour seeks his advancement rather than endeavouring to love him, thus enlarging his soul and allowing the power of his I to flourish. Only when we understand by this the special power of the Yahweh God and consider the way in which he revealed himself to Moses can we understand the distinctive kind of consciousness that is now intended to flow into the people, founded everywhere not on abstract laws but on provisions that are healthy and salutary in the broadest sense for body, soul and spirit. Whoever abides by these commandments not in an abstract but in a living way acts to further the wholesomeness, health and overall advancement of life. At the time they were given, there was no other way to manifest these things than to issue the commandments as decrees that should be followed in a certain way. The other nations lived in a quite different way from the Jewish people, and did not need commandments of this kind, of such meaning and intent.

When studying the Ten Commandments today, our scholars and academics translate them with dictionary in hand and compare them with other laws such as the Law of Hammurabi, and this shows that they have no sense whatever of the presiding impulse at work in them. 'Thou shalt not steal!' or 'Thou shalt sanctify this or that feast day!' are not the important thing. What matters here is the spirit flowing through these Ten Commandments, and how this spirit is connected with the spirit of this people, in whose midst Christianity was created.

If we wish to understand this work of the Ten Commandments at all, we have to sense and feel everything involved in the developing autonomy, the emerging priesthood of each and every member of this people. Today we do not at all live in an age where such things can be experienced so tangibly as the members of the Jewish people experienced them. This is why modern translations impose all kinds of dictionary-derived interpretations that do not correspond to the spirit of the commandments. We read suggestions such as that the Mosaic people emerged from a Bedouin tribe and that therefore the same kind of laws could not be given to them as would be given to a nation of farmers. And this is the reason—academics conclude—why the Ten Commandments must have been given at a later date, and were later attributed to an earlier time. If the Ten Commandments were really what these gentlemen surmise, they would be right. But they do not understand their real origins. It is true that the Jews were originally a kind of Bedouin people. But these commandments were given them so that they could progress through the impulse of I power towards an entirely new era. This is the best demonstration of the fact that nations develop and are formed out of the spirit. One can scarcely imagine a greater prejudice than to say that in Moses' day the Jewish people were a nomadic Bedouin people. What point would there possibly have been then in giving them the Ten Commandments? It was meaningful to give such laws to the Jewish people so that they might be informed as strongly as possible by the I impulse. This people received the Ten Commandments so as to give their outward life an entirely new form— because an entirely new kind of life was to be created out of the spirit.

The Ten Commandments thus exerted an ongoing influence, and this is why insightful early Christians also refer to the Law of Moses. They see how the I impulse is changed through the Mystery of Golgotha from what it was at the time of Moses. They acknowledge that the I impulse is deeply imbued with the spirit of the Ten Commandments and that the people grew strong when they adhered to these laws. Now though, they say, something new has come. Now we have the figure upon whom the Mystery of Golgotha is founded. Now this I can gaze upon what passed in such hidden form through the ages—upon the greatest aspect it can acquire, rendering it strong and powerful as it seeks to emulate the one who suffered at Golgotha, who is the greatest exemplar for the future of evolving humanity. For those, therefore, who really understood Christianity, Christ replaced the impulses that worked in a preparatory way in the Old Testament.

And thus we see that there truly is a deeper way to view the Ten Commandments.

Lecture 10

Berlin, 8 December 1908

ADHERING to our envisaged programme, this winter we will gather a series of apparently widely divergent details relating to human health and sickness and present them in these branch meetings. And at a later stage these details will come together to form a whole, culminating in a specific insight towards which we are gradually working our way. In the first of the relevant lectures in this series,[31] we offered a kind of classification of diseases; and last time[32] we tried to find our way in to what we can really only call the wording of the Ten Commandments. Everything else over and above the actual words will emerge during the next few meetings. Last time we were chiefly concerned to acquaint ourselves with the content and inner orientation of the commandments. Today let us speak about other things which have scarcely any direct connection with preceding and subsequent matters, since they are a collation of details whose over-arching intent will only later become clear.

Initially today we will examine a significant moment in human evolution on earth. Those who have worked for a longer time within the anthroposophical movement have long been familiar with this, while the others will only gradually find their way into these trains of thought.

The moment in human evolution we wish to recall lies a long way back. If we go back through the post-Atlantean period and then through Atlantean times to ancient Lemuria, we encounter the moment when the division into sexes occurs for earthly humanity. As you know, we cannot speak of a division into sexes in the human realm prior to this.

I would like to make it quite clear that we are not now speaking of the very first emergence of two sexes in general in earth evolution, or in our whole process of evolution as it extends to the kingdoms surrounding us. Phenomena that must be assigned to a division into two sexes do emerge earlier. But as far as the human realm is concerned, the division into two sexes only occurs during the Lemurian epoch. Prior to this we find a human form that is very differently configured, and in a sense contains both sexes in an undifferentiated form. We can imagine the outward transition from hermaphrodite existence to a division into two sexes by picturing how the earlier, hermaphrodite human form gradually developed into a group of individuals who developed the characteristics of one gender, the female, in a more pronounced way, while the other group accentuated male characteristics. However, this is still a long way from a division into two genders; it is just an increasing accentuation of one set of characteristics, at a time, also, when humanity still inhabited a very tenuous substantiality.

We have initially brought this period to mind here because our question today focuses on the purpose and meaning of the origin of the two sexes. We can only ask about such a meaning if we stand on a spiritual-scientific foundation, since physical evolution acquires its purpose and significance from higher worlds. As long as we stand in the physical world and also study the physical world with, if you like, a philosophic eye, it is somewhat childlike to speak of 'purpose'. Goethe and others rightly poked fun at those who speak of nature's purposes in a way that suggests, say, that nature in its wisdom produced cork so that man could make stoppers with it. This is a childlike view of things and can only lead to illusion about aspects of key importance. Such an observation would be like looking at a clock and imagining that clever little devils are at work inside it to move the hands forward. If we wish to perceive the real nature of a clock we have to find our way into the mind that made it, that of the clockmaker. And likewise, if we wish to gain insight into the purposeful nature of the world we have to pass beyond its physical properties and enter into the realm of spirit. Thus purpose, meaning and aim are words we can only apply to evolution if we study it from a spiritual-scientific perspective. It is in this sense that we ask now:

What purpose lay in the gradual elaboration of the two genders and their reciprocal interplay?

The purpose will become clear to you if we consider how fertilization, as we know it, which we can also call the mutual influence of the two sexes, previously occurred in a different way. We should not think that the time when the division into two genders occurred was the first instance of what we can call fertilization. That is not so. In the periods preceding a two-gender humanity, though, fertilization occurred quite differently. Looking back with clairvoyant consciousness we find that there was a time in human evolution on earth when fertilization already occurred in connection with nutrition, so that the hermaphrodite entities of earlier times absorbed fertilizing powers along with food. In this period, therefore, when nutrition was of course also a much subtler business, the nutritional juices human beings imbibed at the same time contained something that endowed them with the capacity to bring forth their own kind. Here you have to remember one thing, though: that the nutritional juices drawn from surrounding materiality did not always contain these fertilization fluids, but did so only at quite specific times. This depended on the cyclical alternations that occurred, which we could compare with our own seasonal changes through the course of a year, with climatic changes and so forth. At very specific times, the nutritional juices these hermaphrodite beings drew from the environment also contained fertilizing power.

If we look back still further with clairvoyant perception we find another peculiarity of ancient reproduction. The multiplicity of individual people as we know it today, resulting in different people's individual characteristics—on which is based the diversity of life in our current cycle of humanity—did not exist prior to the emergence of two genders. There was instead a great uniformity. These beings closely resembled each other and also their ancestors. Not yet divided into two genders, they were outwardly similar in appearance, and inwardly too they were all fairly alike in character. The fact that people resembled each other so closely did not have the same disadvantage in those times as it would have for our own. Imagine how boring human life would be if people today were born with the same appearance, and character too. How little could really happen in human life since each person would want the same as every other. This was not so in ancient times. When human beings were more etheric, more spiritual, not so deeply immersed in materiality, people were really very similar at birth and even for a certain period during childhood; and teachers in those days would not have needed to worry about one being a wild tearaway while the other was quiet and retiring. In different eras people were different in character, but basically they were, in a certain sense, very similar to one another. During the course of an individual's life, however, this did not remain so. Through inhabiting a softer, more spiritual corporeality, a person was far more open to prevailing influences arising in his environment, and under these influences he would change enormously during this ancient epoch of the earth. In a sense he became more individualized through having what one might call a soft, malleable nature. Thus he became more or less an imprint of his surroundings. In particular, at a quite specific period of life, which would coincide with puberty today, it became possible for everything in his surroundings to affect him.

The difference between changing periods of time, which we could compare with our alternating seasons today, was very great in those days, and a person's location in a particular place in the world had a major effect on him. In those times, a short journey from one place to another would affect him profoundly. When people go on long journeys today, however much they see and experience they basically return as the same people—unless someone is really extremely susceptible to impressions. In ancient times this was not so: everything exerted the greatest influence on people, and as long as they inhabited this soft materiality I spoke of they could only very gradually become individualized in the course of life. At a certain point this capacity ceased.

A further aspect is that the earth itself became increasingly dense; and as the substance of the earth, its 'earthiness' if you like, became more pronounced, this uniformity came to be harmful. For then people increasingly lost the capacity to change during their lives; instead they were endowed with a great, innate density. And this is also why people today change so little during their lives. This led Schopenhauer[33] to state that basically people cannot change their character at all. This is because they inhabit such dense materiality, and are unable easily to work on it and change it. If we were able to change our limbs, as was still the case in those ancient times, for instance extending or shortening a limb at will, according to need, we would be far more open to impressions. Basically we would then incorporate into our own individuality something that allowed us to make changes within ourselves. A person is always in intimate contact with his surroundings, especially with his social milieu. To ensure we understand each other very precisely, I would like to tell you something you may not have considered, but which is certainly true.

Assume that you are sitting opposite someone and talking to him. I'm not speaking of someone with profound esoteric schooling but of normal, ordinary life and ordinary, interpersonal dialogue. So imagine that two people face each other, one of whom speaks while the other listens. Usually we think that the person listening is not doing anything. That's not the case. In such phenomena we can still see the influence of our surroundings. Although outwardly imperceptible, inwardly it is very clear, and even striking, that the person listening reproduces everything the other does—even movements of the physical vocal cords are imitated so that the listener speaks along with what the other says. Whenever you listen you are speaking along with what you hear, with a slight resonance of your vocal cords and the rest of the speech apparatus. And it makes a great difference whether the person speaking has a grating or a pleasant voice, which you then reproduce with corresponding movements. In this respect we copy everything, and since this basically occurs continuously, it exerts a great influence on all education—albeit only within these narrow parameters.

If you take this vestige we have retained of openness to our surroundings, and expand it to the greatest conceivable scope, you will have an idea of how, in ancient times, people were immersed in and experienced their environment. In those times, for instance the human imitative capacity was developed to a magnificent degree. If one person performed a movement, everyone else did it too. Only in very specific domains do tiny vestiges of this remain nowadays; if one person yawns, for instance, others may yawn too. But remember that in those ancient times a dull, twilight form of consciousness existed. Such an imitative capacity is intrinsically connected with this.

As the earth with everything upon it grew ever denser, human beings grew increasingly unable to reshape themselves under the influence of their environment. For instance, in the Atlantean era, which relatively speaking is not so ancient, a sunrise was something that had a hugely formative effect on human beings since they were so inwardly open to its influence, and this resulted in magnificent inner experiences. When these repeatedly occurred, they altered a person greatly during his lifetime. All this diminished and gradually faded the more humanity advanced.

In Lemurian times, before the moon departed from the earth, a great danger threatened human beings—that of rigidifying entirely, or becoming mummified. The gradual withdrawal of the moon from our earth evolution kept this danger at bay. At the same time as the moon departed, the division into sexes occurred, and this gave a renewed impulse for human individualization. If it had been possible for humanity to reproduce without the two genders, it would not have embarked on this individualization. Today's diversity of humankind is due to the interplay of the sexes. If a solely feminine aspect were at work, human individuality would be extinguished and all people would become the same. Through the additional influence of a masculine aspect, people are endowed with individual characters from birth. The significance of the interplay of the sexes is that emergence and separation of the masculine element enabled individualization from birth onwards to replace the old form of individualization. What the whole environment brought about in former times was concentrated into the reciprocal action of the sexes, thus pushing individualization back to the emergence of the physical human being at birth. This is the purpose of the collaborative interplay between the two genders. Individualization occurs through the effect of the male sex on the female.

But in consequence something else also came into play for human beings. If I describe this now, I beg you to consider it as something absolutely characteristic of humanity: if we stand on the foundations of spiritual science we should not regard such a thing as applying in the same way to animals as to human beings. The subtler forces at work in health and disease are subject to very different causes in animals than in humans. What I am going to say therefore relates exclusively to humankind, and we will first need to become aware of the subtler aspects at work here.

Place yourself back in those ancient times when human beings were entirely given up to their surroundings, which pervaded them. On the one hand the nutritional fluids drawn from the environment also facilitated fertilization, while on the other, human beings were individualized by environmental influences. Standing on the foundation of spiritual science, we know of course that everything surrounding us and affecting us, whether as light, sound, heat, cold, hardness, softness, this colour or that, is the outward expression of something spiritual. And in those ancient times people perceived what was spiritual rather than external sensory impressions. When someone looked up to the sun he did not see the physical globe of the sun but instead what was preserved in the Persian religion as Ahura Mazda, as the 'Great Aura'. The spiritual aspect, the totality of spiritual sun beings appeared to him, and the same was true of air, water and everything in the surrounding environment. Today, if you drink in the beauty of a painting, you can have a sort of distillation of this experience, except that at that time it was richer and more vivid. If we wished to express the ancient outlook, instead of saying, 'This or that tastes like this to me,' we would have to say, 'This or that spirit does me good.' It was like this when people engaged with their surroundings through eating—which was an entirely different kind of activity from nowadays. And the time when fertilization powers were imbibed was likewise quite different: a phenomenon of the spiritual environment. Spirits overshadowed the human being and stimulated him to bring forth his own kind; and this was also experienced and observed as a spiritual process.

Now it became ever more impossible for the human being to see the spiritual aspect of his surroundings. This was increasingly veiled by his day consciousness. Gradually he ceased to perceive the underlying spirit of things, seeing instead only external objects that are the outward expression of the spirit, and forgetting the spirit that stands behind them. And as his form grew ever more dense, the spiritual influences upon him diminished. The process of densification and consolidation rendered human beings increasingly autonomous, separating them off from their spiritual environment. The further back we delve into ancient times, the more divine and spiritual such environmental influence becomes. The human organism was really such that people were a reflection and likeness of their environment, of the spiritual entities hovering around them; they were images of the gods who were present in the ancient eras of the earth.

This faded increasingly, especially through the interplay of the two sexes, which caused the spiritual world to recede from human gaze. Human beings increasingly perceived the sensory world. We must picture this very vividly. Just picture how, in those ancient times, humans were fertilized from the divine-spiritual world. The gods themselves bestowed their powers to make human beings resemble them. This meant that what we call illness did not exist in those ancient times. There was no inner disposition or susceptibility to illness—there could not be since everything in the human being, and everything working upon him, came from the sound and healthy divine-spiritual cosmos. Divine-spiritual entities are healthy, and at that time they formed the human being in their image; and so the human being was healthy too. But as he approached the time when the interplay of the sexes began, along with the withdrawal of spiritual worlds, and became individualized, the health of divine-spiritual entities increasingly receded from him, to be replaced by something else. This reciprocal action of the sexes was, you see, embedded in and accompanied by passions and instincts engendered in the physical world.

We must specifically look for this stimulus originating in the physical world after humankind had reached the point where the two sexes came to please one another, in a physical, sensory way. By no means did this immediately occur the moment the two sexes existed. The effect of the two sexes upon each other—in Atlantean times too—occurred when physical consciousness slumbered really, as it were when everything slept. Only in the middle era of Atlantean times did the pleasure of the two sexes in each other arise, what we can call passionate love—and thus a sensual love that was blended with pure, supersensible love, what we might call 'Platonic love'—an expression scarcely given credence today, but it does really have its place. Platonic love would exist to a much greater extent if sensual love were not mixed up with it. And whereas in the past everything that helped shape humankind was a consequence of the divine-spiritual environment, this was now increasingly replaced by the reciprocal influence of the passions and drives of the two sexes. Sensual desire, stimulated by the outward eye, by external sight of the other gender, became connected with the reciprocal effect of the two sexes. At birth, therefore, something connected with the distinctive nature of passions and feelings in humans embedded in physical life was incorporated into them. Previously human beings received what existed in them from the divine-spiritual beings of their surroundings, but now, through the act of fertilization, they were endowed with something they absorbed from the sensory world and internalized as autonomous, self-contained beings.

After human beings had entered into a two-gender condition, they endowed their offspring with what they themselves had experienced in the world of the senses. So picture two human beings. These two humans live in the physical world, perceiving it through their senses, thereby developing various drives and desires stimulated by external things. Notably they develop drives and passions through their own, outwardly stimulated sensual attraction to each other. What approaches people from without is drawn down into the sphere of autonomous humankind, is no longer in full accord with the divine-spiritual cosmos. This is acquired by human beings through the physical act of fertilization; it is instilled into them. And this mundane life of their own, which they do not derive from divine worlds but from the outward aspect of the divine-spiritual world, is passed on to their offspring through fertilization. If someone is worse in this respect, he passes on worse qualities to his descendants than another who has pure, good qualities.

And thus we have what we must conceive as the authentic meaning of 'original sin'. Original sin arises when human beings acquire the capacity to implant in their descendants their individual experiences in the physical world. Each time the sexes are fired by passion, the constituents of the two sexes are blended into the human souls descending from the astral world. Whenever someone incarnates he descends from the world of devachan and forms his astral sphere in accordance with the distinctive nature of his individuality. This astral sphere merges with something intrinsic to the parents' astral bodies, their drives, passions and desires, and thus a person acquires what his ancestors have experienced. What passes through the generations and is acquired and transmitted as intrinsically human characteristics in the course of generations, is what we must understand by the term 'original sin'. And now we come to something different again—something entirely new entered humanity through human individualization.

In earlier times divine-spiritual beings, who were entirely sound and whole, formed the human being in their image. But now, as autonomous being, the human being sundered himself from the universal harmony of divine-spiritual health. His singularity was, in a certain sense, in opposition to this whole divine-spiritual environment. Imagine that you have a creature that only develops in obedience to environmental influences. It will embody the nature of this environment. But now imagine that it encloses itself in a skin so that it develops its own qualities in addition to those of its environment. When humans became individualized through the division of the sexes, they also developed their own inner characteristics, causing opposition between the great, intrinsically healthy divine-spiritual harmony and individualized human nature. As these individual characteristics continued to take effect, becoming a real factor, human evolution for the first time incorporated a capacity for illness. So here we meet the moment in human evolution where disease first becomes a possibility, connected as it is with human individualization. Prior to this, while humankind was still connected with the divine-spiritual world, disease could not arise. It first arose alongside individualization, at the same time as the division of the sexes. This holds true only of human evolution, and cannot be applied in the same way to the animal world.

Disease is indeed a result of the processes I have just described; and in particular the astral body, basically, was the aspect originally affected in this way. The effect of the two sexes flows into the astral body first incorporated by the human soul as it descends from the world of devachan. The astral body is therefore the part of us that most clearly expresses non-divine nature. The etheric body is already more divine, since we do not exert such a strong influence on it, and most divine of all is the physical body, this temple of God, for it has been thoroughly removed from human influence. In our astral body we seek all kinds of pleasure, and can entertain all possible desires that are harmful for the physical body, but our physical body, by contrast, has been preserved as such a wondrous instrument that it is capable of resisting substances toxic to the heart for decades, as well as other disruptive influences from the astral body. All these processes, we have to say, have rendered the human astral body the worst aspect of our nature. If you study human nature more carefully, you will find that the causes of illness are most deeply rooted in the astral body, and in its harmful effect on the etheric body, and then transmitted via the latter to the physical body. So now we can understand certain things that cannot otherwise be understood. I would now like to speak of ordinary mineral-based medicines.

A medicine derived from the mineral kingdom acts first on the human physical body. What purpose does it have, therefore, for us to treat our physical body with a mineral medicine? Please note that I am not speaking at present of any kind of herbal medicine but of purely mineral constituents—metals, salts and so forth. Let us assume that someone takes a certain mineral medicine. As the clairvoyant gaze observes this, it discovers something very remarkable. Clairvoyant consciousness can accomplish the following feat: it always has the ability to divert attention away from something. You can divert attention away from the whole physical human body, perceiving only the ether body, astral body and I aura. Using strongly negative attention, you can suggest away the physical body. Now if someone takes a mineral medicine of some kind, you can withdraw your whole clairvoyant attention from everything else and direct it solely towards the metal or mineral that is now within him. By suggestion you make the bones, muscles, blood and so forth disappear, and direct your attention solely to the particular mineral substance that has permeated the person. Clairvoyant consciousness then discovers something very remarkable: this mineral substance has been finely distributed throughout so that it assumes the human form. Before you stands a human form—a human phantom—consisting of the substance that the person has ingested. Let us assume that he took antimony. Then you see before you a human form consisting of finely distributed antimony; and the same would be true of every ingested mineral medicine. You make a new human within yourself, consisting of this mineral substance. You incorporate it into you. So now let us ask what purpose this might have, and what point.

The point is as follows. If you left as he is someone who needs something like this, and did not give him the medicine despite his real need of it, certain negative forces in his astral body would work upon his ether body, and the ether body in turn on the physical body, gradually destroying it. Now, though, you have imbued the physical body with a double whose effect is to prevent the physical body from hearkening to the astral body's influence. Imagine a bean plant; if you give it a supporting cane, it winds around it and now no longer follows the movements of the wind. This double acts as a kind of cane for a person, formed from the incorporated substance. It keeps the physical body intact and withdraws it from the influences of the astral body and ether body. By this means you render a person's physical body independent in a sense from his astral and ether body. That is the effect of a mineral medicine. But you will also immediately see the negative aspect of this, for it does indeed have a very deleterious side to it. Since you have artificially removed the physical body from its connection with the other bodies, weakening the influence of astral and ether body on the physical body, you have made the physical body independent—and the more you administer such medicines to your body the less the astral and ether bodies will engage with it. Thus the physical body will grow to be inwardly hardened, an autonomous entity subject to its own laws.

Imagine what people are doing, what the effect on their body is, when they take various mineral medicines throughout their life. Someone who has gradually absorbed a great many mineral medicines bears the phantom of these minerals within him—a dozen such mineral medicines perhaps. These enclose the physical body within four walls as it were. How then can the astral body and ether body engage with it? Such a person actually drags his physical body around with him and is fairly powerless in relation to it. Someone who has medicated himself in this way for a long time will find, if he seeks a more psychological form of treatment that acts particularly on the subtler bodies, that he has become more or less unreceptive to soul influences. He has rendered his physical body independent and denied it the capacity to allow what could occur in the subtler bodies to work through into the physical body. And this has happened particularly because he bears so many phantoms in himself that do not act in harmony—one pulling him one way, the other another. In denying himself the possibility of acting upon the body from his soul-spiritual aspects, he should not be surprised if a spiritually-based cure has little success. Whenever a curative influence from the soul is involved, therefore, it is important to remember what kind of person stands before you. Has he put his astral body or ether body out of action by rendering the physical body independent? If so, it will be very difficult to help him with a spiritual cure.

We can now understand how mineral substances act on the human being. They engender doubles in him that preserve his physical body and remove him from potentially harmful effects of his astral or ether body. Today, almost all our medicine is geared to this, since materialistic medicine is unaware of the human being's subtler bodies, and only knows how to treat the physical body in some fashion.

Today we have considered the effects of mineral substances. We will need also to speak of the effects on the human organism of the healing forces available in herbal medicines, as well as those of animal substances. Then we will pass on to the influences, the means of healing, that can exist in the interpersonal soul realm and are thus spiritual. You will see, however, that it is necessary for our sequence of observations to first appraise and properly understand concepts such as 'original sin'. Today people so easily overlook certain things and fail to understand them.

LECTURE 11

BERLIN, 21 DECEMBER 1908

W E can only ascend to ever higher domains in these meetings here by arranging the courses running parallel to these branch lectures as we have done.[34] I would therefore ask you to take note of these courses as far as you can. We have to have a place where we can advance further with the lectures—otherwise we would have to start again anew each year.

Today we will examine something that again, apparently, is worlds away from preceding lectures, but which will connect with the whole context of this year's studies. I would like to pick up on a remark in one of the recent public lectures, the one on 'Superstition from a spiritual-scientific perspective'.[35] There I made a comment that cannot be further developed in a public lecture since background knowledge is required to delve more deeply into it. Such knowledge draws not so much on intellectual acuity as on a capacity for insight founded on our whole constitution of soul, which we can acquire through long years of involvement in anthroposophical branch life. It is only through such patient labours that we can succeed in regarding as possible and probable what we would previously have dismissed as absurd, by taking it with us into our lives and seeing to what extent it holds true. The remark I would like to start from was this: It is a common fact, and not a superstition, that in certain illnesses such as pneumonia the seventh day of illness represents a crisis. This invariably occurs on the seventh day, and is the point when a patient may die, and when the physician must take great pains to help him survive the crisis. Every sensible physician acknowledges this—but physicians cannot study the causes of it since they have no idea of underlying spiritual realities. Let us first establish the fact that something remarkable occurs here and is connected with the mysterious number seven.

We need to study the human being in a way that offers us insight into this and diverse other realities. You all know—for I have referred to it here on countless occasions—that we can only gain insight into the human being if we understand him to be constituted of four aspects— physical body, ether body, astral body and I. These four aspects of human nature have the most varied interrelationships and interactions. Every aspect works upon the other and thus they have a whole interpenetrating context. But this interaction is very complex. Only very slowly and gradually can we gain insight into these connections, and likewise into the way they relate to certain forces, processes and entities in the whole cosmos. By virtue of all the aspects of our being we exist in a continual and—likewise very important—alternating connection with the cosmos. What we perceive as physical body, ether body, and so forth, is interconnected but at the same time connected with the cosmos too—with the whole world that spreads out around us. You see, what we contain within us is also in a sense outside us; and so we will best perceive these inner and outer relationships if we observe the human being in the two states of sleeping and waking.

When we see a person asleep, we have the physical and ether bodies lying in the bed; and outside these two, in a sense, are the astral body and I. However, this is somewhat inaccurate. A certain lack of precision will suffice for many things, but today let us examine these realities more carefully. The astral body and the I are, then, initially not active within the body. The physical body with its nervous and vascular system, and the ether body cannot however exist at all unless imbued by an astral body and some form of I configuration. The ether body, too, could not exist without higher beings imbuing it. The moment we rise out with our own astral body and I, a replacement is needed to accomplish the activities of these two aspects of human nature. The human body cannot lie there without having an I and astral body active within it, so that when asleep, too, we still need an active astral body and I. But to be accurate we ought to put it like this: the I and the astral body active in a person's sleeping physical body are also present during the day, but then their activity is undermined by his own astral body and I, whose activity renders that of the other, higher beings null and void.

If we try to picture the I as it lives in us today in a waking state, we can say that this human I dwells within the human body while we are awake and during this time its activity removes its sphere of action from an all-encompassing, universal I. What does this restricted I of ours actually do during sleep? It is really fairly accurate to say that having emancipated itself during the day from the great universal I and, having lived in the human body by its own devices, it is immersed during the night in the universal I and gives itself up to its own intrinsic activity. It is precisely by virtue of this immersion, this sinking of the day I into the universal I, that the universal I can work unhindered, and can sweep away the substances of tiredness accumulated by the day I. The full compass of the night I becomes possible through the immersion and submersion of the day I in the universal I. If you wish to conceive this pictorially, you can see this relationship between the day I and the night I as if the former described a circle whose larger portion represents the time spent outside the great I—in which it is only submerged during the night. It may be outside for 16 hours for instance, and immersed in the night I for eight hours.

You will only properly understand this if you attend seriously to what I have just said, that your I never remains the same during the 16 hours—if we assume this to be the normal waking period—and that during this time the I undergoes continual changes, and it describes one part of a circle, then is submerged and also undergoes changes during the night of which people are ordinarily unaware. These changes pass increasingly into the unconscious until a culmination is reached, and then the I slowly becomes more conscious again. In the course of 24 hours, therefore, the human I continually undergoes certain changes like a clock hand describing a circle, and from time to time submerging itself in the great universal I.

Our astral body also undergoes changes in a very similar way. The astral body alters in a way that can also be symbolically conceived as a circle. In the astral body likewise the changes are such that we must, in a sense, speak of submersion in a universal astral body. Nowadays, though, people no longer notice this submersion in a universal astral body. In former times they certainly did notice it. In those days you can say that people felt an alternation between their own deeply intrinsic astral feelings at one moment and quite different feelings at another. At one point a person experienced the outer, surrounding world more vividly, at another, by contrast, he felt his own inner life more strongly. People were therefore able to perceive very different nuances in the astral body's mode of feeling. This is because the astral body undergoes rhythmic alternations in the course of seven days—thus seven times 24 hours—which can again be compared with a circular motion. Just as the I undergoes rhythmic changes in a period of 24 hours, still expressed today in the alternation between sleeping and waking, so the astral body does this in seven times 24 hours. Such rhythmic changes occurred in a very vital way in primeval human beings. Thus rhythmic alternations occur in the astral body over the course of seven days, and from the eighth day onwards the rhythm repeats. During part of this rhythmic periodicity, the astral body indeed immerses itself in a general, universal astral body. The rest of the time it remains more outside this universal astral body. This can give you a sense that what appears in us as general astral body and general I while we are asleep has great importance for our life. The I in which we immerse ourselves in sleep, which keeps our blood pulsing at night, is the same as that which works in our body during sleep.

If we sleep during the day, too, we immerse ourselves in this general I, thus introducing a certain irregularity into our rhythm which would have had a destructive effect in former times. Today it is no longer so destructive since, in this respect, human life has significantly altered in our own times. During a seven-day period, the human astral body really is submerged in the same part of the general, universal astral body that penetrates the physical body and ether body during sleep. Inner feelings and emotions change in consequence. Today scarcely any attention is paid to this, whereas formerly it simply could not be ignored.

However, besides the I and the astral body, the ether body also undergoes quite specific rhythmic changes. Symbolically speaking, the human ether body turns on its axis once in four times seven days, returning to the same processes after this period as on the first day of the cycle. A quite specific rhythm occurs here in four times seven days; and we enter a realm here that we would need to speak about in more detail to make it all comprehensible. You will recall me saying that the man's ether body is female, while the woman's is male. The rhythm is not the same for a male and female ether body, but we will not go into this today. I would just like to stress the fact that such a rhythm occurs, and approximately—because of the difference between man and woman—does so in four times seven days.

This is not all, though. Quite specific processes also recur rhythmically in the physical body, however improbable this may seem to people today. Nowadays they have almost entirely faded since we ought to become independent of certain processes, but the clairvoyant observer can detect them. If the physical body were left entirely to its own devices, this rhythm would unfold in ten times seven times four (280) days in the woman, and twelve times seven times four (336) days in the man. This would happen if we were given over entirely to the intrinsic laws of our rhythms. It used to be so, but we have grown freer from surrounding cosmic influences. Thus we have processes that recur rhythmically in the four aspects of the human being. Each of the rhythms can be pictured, if you like, as a cycle. Today, of course, the rhythm we would accomplish in our physical body if it were left entirely to its own devices only approximately coincides with purely spatial, external physical processes corresponding to this rhythm. These relationships to the cosmos have altered due to compression of our organism in a way that furthers human freedom.

The numbers ten times seven times four, or twelve times seven times four, will have shown you that the rhythm of the physical body relates roughly to the cycle of the year. You can understand these changes to the outward physical body in symbolic form if you picture a person revolving during the course of a year, and being on the near side of the sun at one point, and on the far side at another. If we conceive him as always looking with his face towards the sun, he will revolve once around himself and once around the sun during the course of a year. Someone who considers this in a solely external way will regard it as a matter of complete indifference, but it is actually very important.

The rhythm occurring here in the four bodies was implanted in us over long, long ages; and the fact that the different bodies can mutually affect each other was ordained by the hierarchies of beings of whom we have often spoken. We know that we are embedded in higher beings. The workings of these spiritual beings whose deeds penetrate physical and spiritual space, engendered these specific relationships. But in considering what has been said now you approach from a different perspective an idea that we often touched on last winter. The rhythm of the physical body began to be established on old Saturn. Incorporation of the ether body in such a way as to harmonize the rhythms of etheric body and physical body originates in the engendering of this rhythm by other spirits, the sun spirits. The interplay of these different rhythms gives rise to a relationship in the same way that the relationship between the two hands of a clock is determined by their rhythm. On old Moon a further rhythm was incorporated, that of the astral body.

Now the spirits who ordained and coordinated our whole cosmos— for all physical reality is an expression of these beings—were obliged to configure external physical movement in correspondence with their inner nature. The fact that the earth orbits the sun once during a year originates in the rhythm implanted in the physical body long before this physical constellation existed. The spatial nature of these heavenly spheres was determined by spiritual realities. The moon orbits the earth in four times seven days because its cycle is intended to correspond to the cycle of the human etheric body, whose rhythm was to find expression in the moon's movement. The changing illumination of the moon by the sun, the four quarters of the moon, corresponds to the different rhythms of the astral body, while the daily revolving of the earth corresponds to the rhythm of the I. Precisely in the rhythm of the I we can discover something that all spiritual science has always taught, yet will strike modern human beings as dreams and fantasy—but is nevertheless true. In primeval times the earth did not turn on its axis. This axial rotation only arose over time. When humanity was still in a different condition on earth, this motion did not yet exist. It was not the earth that was first stimulated to rotate but the human being himself. The spirits to whom the human being is subject stimulated the I to rotate; and the human I then, in fact, took this earth with it and rotated it around itself. The earth's rotation results from the I rhythm. However astonishing this sounds, it is still true. First the human being's spiritual aspects, developing towards the I, had to receive the impetus to rotate, and then they took the earth with them. Later this changed of course. The human being became free on earth and conditions altered such that the human being became free of surrounding cosmic powers. But this is how he was originally. So you see how all physical reality around us is really an emanation of spirit. The spirit is the *primum mobile*, and from it flow all conditions and spatial relationships in the world.

And now consider the astral body for a moment. In the course of seven days you can say that it accomplishes a cycle. Consider how diseases are connected with certain irregularities of the astral body, and that they arise when some such irregularity reverberates through the ether body and reaches the physical body. Now let us assume that the astral body has some intrinsic defect. Through this defect it works upon the ether body, and thus the defect is replicated and carried through into the physical body. Then the latter also becomes defective, and the organism begins to revolt against the defect, activating defensive forces. Fever is the most common form of revolt and invokes our healing powers. Fever is not illness, but a state in which we summon all the powers that exist everywhere in our organism to remedy this defect. This revolt of the whole organism against the defect is usually expressed in fever. Fever is the most beneficial, most healing factor in disease. The part of the body that has become defective cannot heal itself and needs to be aided by powers originating elsewhere—and this comes to expression in fever.

Now picture a fever accompanying pneumonia. Something or other has harmed the lungs. Particularly when the human lungs suffer harm of some kind, the astral body is implicated as the original sufferer of harm. This defect then passes through the ether body and is transmitted to the physical body. The original cause of pneumonia always lies in the astral body, and there is no other way in which this disease arises. Now consider the rhythm of the astral body. On the day when pneumonia appears, the astral body works upon the physical body. The body starts to revolt in the form of fever. After seven days the astral body and ether body are once again in the same reciprocal position, so that parts of each encounter one another again. But the astral body does not meet the same part of the ether body since, in the meantime, the latter has undergone its own rhythm. Instead the astral body meets a subsequent part of it, which it in turn affects and influences; and in fact this other part of the ether body is affected in an opposite way. Now the fever is suppressed. Since the part of the astral body that coincided seven days ago with the preceding quarter of the ether body now coincides with its next quarter, the opposite process to what occurred seven days ago is induced—that is, the reaction to the fever. The opposite rhythm of the body suppresses the fever again. You see, the human body exists in order to be healthy, and this is the purpose of rhythm. In the first seven days certain effects surface and in the following seven days they must lapse. When we are healthy there is an alternation between this rising and falling rhythm. But when we are ill, suppression of fever represents a life-threatening danger. Whereas in healthy people a rising process is reversed on the seventh day, this rising process needs to be maintained in a sick person. But the vehement rise causes a vehement fall—and this is what causes the crisis on the seventh day of pneumonia.

We can understand this if we consider that the lungs formed at a time when the moon had already separated from the earth and was preparing to develop its rhythm; and when our day rhythm was also starting to develop. This is why the lungs today are still connected with the astral body and the rhythm of the ether body.

Thus you see how spiritual science can illumine abnormal conditions in human life, and how the whole nature of the human being can be recognized if we grasp these connections. This is why the sciences will only become productive again if people engage fully with the great discoveries of spiritual science. In former times—roughly up to the middle of our evolution on earth—all human rhythms were in much greater harmony with the external rhythms of nature. Since then—that is, since the middle of the Atlantean period—everything has shifted and become transposed. Our inner nature has emancipated itself from external rhythms. Within, we have retained our old rhythm. Precisely through the lack of accord between rhythms, we have acquired independence and freedom—otherwise the development towards freedom would not have been possible in humanity's history. The human rhythm has overtaken that of the sun, or of the earth as it relates to the sun. Something similar is true of the other rhythms, for instance that of the astral body. In former times the human being experienced very diverse nuances of mood through the seven-day cycle. For some of the time, everything external made a great impression on him while for another period he lived more inwardly. Since these rhythms no longer accord with each other today, states of inner experience are retained during the period when a person takes more pleasure in the external world, and vice versa. They become intermeshed and balance each other out; and the astral body, you can say, becomes 'well tempered' in consequence, in the musical sense. In people who live more in their astral body, subtle observation can allow us to perceive such fluctuations of mood or sentiment. In the case of people suffering from mental illness, we can identify differences in the astral body's states.

The rhythm of the I arose latest, but here too things shift and become interfused. We can of course sleep during the day and be awake at night. But in former times this rhythm always accorded with the external one. In Atlantis it would have been very harmful if human beings had tried to sleep during the day and be awake at night—this would have caused havoc in their lives. Today the rhythm has been retained to some extent, but has emancipated itself from the external one. It is just like setting an accurate clock precisely to solar time—you can then read off solar hours precisely. But now imagine that at seven in the evening you set the clock to twelve—the clock's rhythm will be correctly retained but will be shifted in relation to the sun. The same is true of us. The ancient rhythm in which we were previously connected with the cosmos has been retained, but has shifted or been transposed. If the clock were a living being, it would be right for it to extricate its rhythm from surrounding rhythms.

In a far-distant future, we must reach the point in our inner evolution of again allowing our rhythm to flow into the world's external reality. Just as there were once beings whose rhythms gave rise to the emergence from them of the movements of sun, moon and earth, so eventually we will transpose our rhythm back into the world once we have attained the stage of divine being. This is the purpose of emancipation from rhythms around us, and here too we can sense the deeper foundations of astrology. But this is not our theme now. Today we just wish to demonstrate that spiritual science is not a sum of abstract ideas for someone egotistically preoccupied with them, but that it will shine a light into the most mundane realities of everyday life. But then we have to have the will to pass from external phenomena to underlying, primary foundations. Rhythm was implanted in matter by the spirit. Today we bear rhythm in us as the legacy of our spiritual origins. However, we can only gain insight into the significance of this rhythm for us, and also for other natural creatures, if we trace it back to primeval conditions. In animals we already find very different interrelationships of the separate aspects—physical body, ether body, astral body and group I. A different rhythm holds good in every species. It is more or less the same for the physical body, but quite distinct rhythms unfold in the ether and astral bodies of the various animals. In a way similar to external categories based on morphology, we can classify animal species according to these different rhythms, depending on how the rhythm of the astral body relates to that of the ether body.

Do not imagine that these rhythms have never been clearly acknowledged. We will be able to show that it is not all that long ago that people had at least a dim awareness of them. Those observant of such things can find calendars used in rural areas with rules for certain relationships between beasts and the land. In former times, a farmer would organize his whole agricultural work in adherence to such rules. And an awareness of such rhythms was spun as a hidden strand into agricultural know-how. Such things can show us that an age of abstraction, of external science, has arisen since the fifteenth and sixteenth centuries—a science whose proponents are no longer able to go to the root of things. This is particularly true in medicine. All we have left here is a kind of fumbling, while the real roots of pathology and therapy delve back into very ancient times. I experienced a martyrdom of the intellect and feelings when phenacetin was tried out. This kind of empirical trial—with no guiding idea—shows that loss of the spirit has also deprived science of real seriousness. We must acquire this seriousness again through spiritual insight. We must certainly learn to distinguish where science presents distorted pictures or where it offers knowledge founded on the spirit. If we inscribe this into our soul we will see how necessary spiritual-scientific insight is, and how it must penetrate all areas of study and life.

LECTURE 12

TODAY we will discuss certain deeply esoteric matters. As strange as it may initially sound, our theme will be 'Mephistopheles and earthquakes'. Besides casting light on a profound esoteric realm when we study the problem of Mephistopheles, we will find that examining the question of earthquakes from a spiritual standpoint is also particularly illuminating. On various occasions, and here too, I have spoken of the earth's interior,[36] thus also touching on the question of earthquakes. Today we will look at this from another perspective, and then discover how what comes to the fore today merges with what has previously been said in earlier lectures about the earth's interior in relation to these extremely tragic events of our earth's crust.

The figure of Mephistopheles, our starting point today, is one you all know from Goethe's drama *Faust*. You know that this Mephistopheles figure is a spiritual being—though today we will not discuss to what extent the poetic guise corresponds to esoteric realities. You will recall that this figure appears in Goethe's *Faust* to tempt and seduce Faust who, in a sense, can be seen as an archetype of someone striving for the heights. In my lectures on Goethe[37] I have characterized the spiritual perspective presented in the scene of Faust's entry to the 'Realm of the Mothers', in which Mephistopheles holds in his hand the key to open the passage to deep underground realms, where the 'Mothers' are to be found. Mephistopheles himself cannot enter this realm. He merely indicates that it is one where 'below' is the same as 'above': 'Sink down then; I might also say: Rise up!'[38] Both would signify the same for this mysterious domain. We also know that Mephistopheles refers to it as one for which he uses the word 'nothing'. In a sense therefore he represents the spirit who regards the void, or nothing, as of no value to him in this realm. Faust replies, as someone today who seeks the spirit would reply to a materialist: 'Within this nothing may I discover all!'[39]

Goethe researchers—such a field of study does exist—have made all kinds of efforts to decipher this figure. In other lectures, too, I have indicated that the etymology of the name 'Mephistopheles' can be found in Hebrew, where *mephiz* means 'obstructor' or 'corrupter', and *tophel* means 'liar'. The name must therefore be seen as a combination of someone who, on the one hand, brings corruption and obstruction to human beings and, on the other, is a figure of deception and illusion—the spirit of untruth.

An attentive reading of the introduction to Goethe's *Faust*, the 'Prologue in Heaven', will discover a resonant phrase there which in a sense reverberates through millennia. At the beginning of his *Faust*, Goethe echoes words from the Book of Job, spoken between God and Job. You need only read this book and you will find that Job lives a good, pious life, and that the sons of the God of light gather before God, amongst them a certain enemy of the light and of the highest God. This enemy of the light states that he has wandered through many lands and has sought and attempted various things. Then God asks him, 'Knowest thou my servant Job?' And the enemy of light—as we will call him for now—replies that he does know him, and he would be able to draw him away from the path of righteousness and corrupt him. You will remember that this spirit must twice attempt to approach Job, that he gets a purchase on him by ruining his outer physical body. He expressly says to God that Job will not be brought to ruin through depriving him of his possessions, but by striking at his flesh and bone. The words in *Faust*, in the Prologue in Heaven when God calls to Mephistopheles, 'Knowest thou Faust? ... My servant' will inevitably recall that biblical passage. And then, in the riposte of Mephistopheles, in words comparable to the Book of Job, one hears the God-opposing spirit say he will be able to 'lead Faust by the nose' and divert him from 'so-called paths of goodness' that lead into the world. In other words, tones separated by millennia here resonate in harmony together.

Whenever you have encountered the figure of Mephistopheles you may have wondered who he really is. And grave errors are made here, which can only be remedied by deeper esoteric insight. The fact that Mephistopheles can be identified with the devil is indicated in the name already, since *tophel* is cognate with 'devil'. But the other question is this—and here we enter a domain fraught with possible errors often made in interpretations of the figure of Mephistopheles: Can he be identified with the spirit we know as Lucifer, of whom we have often spoken in relation to humanity's evolutionary history? During the Lemurian age, and subsequently, this spirit approached humanity with his hosts, and intervened in human evolution in a certain way. In Europe people tend to conflate Mephistopheles, as he figures in Goethe's *Faust*—but also as he has appeared in all forms of folk literature, in puppet plays and so forth—with Lucifer. In these traditions we repeatedly encounter the figure of Mephistopheles, and must ask whether this figure and his fellows are the same as the figure and fellows of Lucifer. In other words, is the mephistophelian influence on us the same as the original luciferic influence? This is the question we will address today.

We know of course when Lucifer approached human beings. We have studied human evolution on earth during the period when the sun with its beings separated from the earth, and then also when the moon separated from the earth along with forces that would have prevented our progress. And we have seen that at a time when the human being was not yet developed enough to enable his astral body to work towards a state of independence, Lucifer and his hosts approached him with, you can say, a double-edged sword. Towards the end of the Lemurian age, the human astral body was exposed to influences derived from Lucifer. If Lucifer had not approached us, we would have remained safe from certain kinds of harm, yet we would not have acquired what we must count among humanity's greatest blessings.

We can clarify the significance of Lucifer's influence if we ask what would have happened if there had been no luciferic influence since Lemurian times, with human evolution remaining at a far remove from Lucifer and the beings associated with him. If that had been the case we would have remained, right into the middle of Atlantean times, subject in all impulses of our astral body, in all its motives, to the influences of certain spiritual beings standing above the human being. It would therefore have taken us far, far longer to direct our capacities of perception and enquiry towards the sensory world, so that during the Lemurian period and the first part of the Atlantean period no desires or passions would have grown within us from sensory perceptions. We would have remained innocent, you can say, in relation to the sensory world, and in everything we did we would have hearkened to the impulses implanted in us by higher beings. Our actions would not have been driven by instinct like that of higher animals today, but by a spiritualized instinct. Every action we took on earth would have been instigated not by merely sensory impulses but by a kind of spiritual instinct. But under Lucifer's influence humans were quicker to say, 'I enjoy this, it attracts me,' or 'This repels me.' They began to follow their own impulses sooner than they would otherwise have done, to become autonomous beings, and develop a degree of inner freedom. This gave rise to a certain human detachment from the world of spirit. To put it quite clearly one can say that without this influence of Lucifer the human being would have remained a spiritualized animal, whose form would gradually have evolved, becoming still more noble and beautiful than the human being did under Lucifer's influence.

The human being would have remained much more angelic if this luciferic influence had not arisen in Lemurian times. On the other hand, though, higher beings would have guided him by spiritual reins. Then, in the middle of the Atlantean period, something new would suddenly have approached him. His eyes would have opened fully so that he perceived the tapestry of the whole physical-sensory world. But he would have seen these surroundings with a divine-spiritual reality standing behind every physical thing—a world of divine, spiritual depths. Until that point, in his dependent state within the lap of God from which he had emerged, he would have looked back to see the gods of light who governed and guided him working upon him and shining into his soul. It is not just a metaphor but really does very much correspond to reality to say that then a new condition would have arisen when he saw around him the full, palpable world of the senses. Yet this sensory world would have appeared to him as transparent, behind which appeared other divine, spiritual beings to replace those he had left behind him. One spiritual world would have closed behind him while a new one opened before him. The human being would have remained a child in the palm of higher, divine, spiritual beings, and autonomy would not have instilled itself in his soul.

Instead of this, of course, Lucifer approached the human being and as it were drew a veil over part of the backdrop of the spiritual world, making it invisible. For as passions, instincts and desires arose in the human astral body, the spiritual beings who had always previously been perceived as standing behind the human being in the world from which he had originated were obscured. This is also why, in the great oracle centres I spoke of last time,[40] primeval Atlantean initiates underwent preparation for perceiving the part of the spiritual world that had been obscured by Lucifer's influence. All preparations by guardians and pupils of the ancient oracle of the Atlantean mysteries were aimed at gazing into this light-filled world of spirit which had withdrawn from human beings due to Lucifer's influence on the human astral body. And then there also appeared the forms we can observe in various soul states that run parallel with initiation, which play into our world from a world of light and dress themselves in the garment the astral world can bestow on them.

The Atlantean initiate in these ancient oracles saw in spirit the figures who rightly appeared to him as higher spiritual beings, who had not descended as far as the physical world and who therefore, when humankind gained a foothold on the earth prematurely, remained invisible to ordinary vision. But it was inevitable that Lucifer himself, in a sense an opponent of these worlds of light, then also became visible to these initiates. The hosts of Lucifer were generally visible to the Atlanteans who—in twilight states of clairvoyant consciousness, in states of sleep and intermediate states between sleeping and waking— could find their way into the higher world of spirit. Whenever human beings gained access to a part of the world of light, at the same time they also perceived a part of the world opposed to it: not Lucifer himself but his fellows. And the enchanting, magnificent sublimity of the astral colours of the light world's forms and figures was equalled by the ter rible, ghastly appearance of the figures who belonged to the opposing world of the tempter.

This influence of Lucifer therefore entered human evolution, and to it we owe our capacity for error and evil—but also our freedom. If this luciferic influence had not arisen, then what I described a moment ago would have occurred in the middle of Atlantean times: the tapestry of the sensory world would have spread before us, with its minerals, plant and animal kingdoms becoming visible to our senses. The world of natural phenomena would have appeared to our sensory perception— thunder and lightning, clouds and air. Atmospheric phenomena would have become fully visible to the outward eye. Yet standing unmistakably behind them we would have perceived the divine beings of spirit who were to permeate and influence us. But the influence of Lucifer had taken effect, and the human being's astral body had previously absorbed this influence. Therefore, from Lemurian times onwards through into Atlantean times, we prepared our physical body in a way that enabled it to become the instrument for directly engaging with the tapestry of the sensory-physical world—which would otherwise have unfolded before us with the spiritual world visible behind it. And so the human being could not immediately perceive the physical world of the senses in the form it would have appeared to him if seen as simultaneously spiritual. The world of the three kingdoms of nature standing lower than the human realm approached him. The physical world dawned on him as one that veiled and obscured the spiritual world like a thick blanket. Thus people could no longer look through it into the spiritual world— and basically this remains true to this day.

Due to the fact that we took this evolutionary course, however, another influence, from a quite different direction, made itself felt in the middle of the Atlantean era. And this is not one we should confuse with that of Lucifer and his hosts. Although Lucifer was the one who first rendered us capable of subjection to this other influence by inducing our physical body to grow more dense and solid than it would otherwise have been. Nevertheless it was a different influence that led us entirely into the sensory, physical world, thus completely closing off the world of spiritual beings from us and locking us out of it. Humankind was led into the illusion that no other world exists than the physical, sensory one unfolding here before us. From the middle of Atlantean times a quite different adversary from Lucifer approached humankind: the one who,

we can say, fogs and obscures human faculties of perception and cognition so that people do not exert themselves, do not develop the
impetus to reach beyond the secrets of the sensory world. If you imagine
that the sensory world became a thick veil under Lucifer's influence,
obscuring the spiritual world behind it, then the influence of this second
being turned the physical world into a thick rind sundering itself from
the spiritual world. And therefore, once again, it was only through
practice and preparation that Atlantean initiates were able to penetrate
this dense physical-sensory curtain.

We first encounter the powers that approached humankind in order
to obscure his view of the other, divine aspect of existence, in the great
teachings given by Zarathustra, leader and figurehead of the ancient
Persian people, to his adherents and faithful followers. It was Zarathustra who had the mission of spreading a culture very different from
that of ancient India. The latter was naturally disposed to yearn for a
past experience of the world of spirit. By contrast, Zarathustra's mission
was to spread amongst a specific people a culture directed towards the
world of the senses, towards mastering the tangible physical world with
the cultural means that could only be established by human exertions in
the external sensory realm of the physical world. This is why ancient
Persian culture was less exposed to the luciferic influence than to that of
the figure who approached humankind from the middle of Atlantean
times onwards and induced a large number of initiates of the time to be
attracted to black magic. This tempter seduced them into misusing
what had become available to them from the world of spirit in service of
the tangible physical world. This immense influx of black magic powers,
which ultimately led to the downfall of Atlantis, has its origin in
temptations emanating from the figure of Ahriman, or Angra Mainyu
who, as Zarathustra taught his people, opposes the bright sun god
known as the Great Aura, or Ahura Mazda.

These two figures, Lucifer and Ahriman, must be clearly distinguished. Lucifer, you see, is a being who, after the sun departed from
the earth, took a different path from the host of spiritual and heavenly
beings. Ahriman, by contrast, is a figure who had already sundered
himself prior to the sun's departure, and assembles quite different forces
in himself. By working upon humankind in Lemurian times, Lucifer

harmed the human being only in respect of the influence on air and water forces that the human being still retained in Atlantean times. You know from my book on the Akashic records (*Cosmic Memory*) that in Atlantean times people still had access to seed potencies contained in plants and animals, and were able to draw these forth in the same way that people today draw powers from coal that they use for steam power to drive their machines. And I have said that if such powers are extracted or drawn out, then they have a mysterious relationship to the natural forces in wind, weather and so forth; and if human beings use these powers in a way opposed to divine intentions, then these forces of nature can be unleashed against them.

This led to the great flood of Atlantis, and the devastating natural forces responsible for the downfall and submergence of the whole Atlantean continent. But already previously to this, humankind no longer had command over the forces of fire and over the connection between these and certain secret forces of the earth. A certain type of interplay between fire and earth was already withdrawn from human command at an earlier stage. But now, through the influence of Ahriman and his cohorts, the human being in a sense regained power over earth and fire forces, doing so in a way which spelled ruin. Much of what we hear about the use of fire in ancient Persia is connected with what I am saying now: diverse forces invoked as black magic, and connected with it, lead people to acquire quite different powers, gaining them influence over fire and earth, and causing mighty and devastating effects. The descendants of the Atlanteans could still have practised black magic in ancient Persia if Zarathustra had not taught them about the adversarial actions of Ahriman towards humanity, as a being who ensnared them and obscured their vision of what ought to emerge as true spiritual power behind the world of the senses. We see therefore that a great deal of post-Atlantean culture—taking its lead from Zarathustra and his followers—was informed, on the one hand, by teachings about the influence of the sublime sun god to whom human beings can turn and, on the other, about the corrupting power of Ahriman and his cohorts.

This Ahriman influences us in the most manifold ways. I have spoken to you of the grandeur of the moment in world evolution when the event of Golgotha occurred. Christ appeared in the world which we enter after death. In this world the influence of Ahriman was far greater still than in the world we see here between birth and death. In the world we pass through between death and a new birth, the influences of Ahriman upon us worked with frightful force and power. If nothing else had happened, then in our passage between death and a new birth humankind would gradually have become shrouded in darkness in what the Greeks rightly felt to be the realm of shades or shadows. And infinite isolation and accentuation of human egotism would have developed in the life between death and a new birth. On being reincarnated, we would have been born into our lives in a way that would have made us crass and terrible egotists. It is therefore more than merely metaphorical to say that after the event of Golgotha, at the moment when blood ran from Christ's wounds, Christ appeared in the world beyond, in the realm of shades, and laid Ahriman in chains. While Ahriman's influence remained, and though all materialistic thinking is basically attributable to him and can only be paralysed if we fully absorb the event of Golgotha, this event nevertheless became the source of strength we draw on to gain entry once more to the divine world of spirit.

This is how Ahriman first rose before human perception—as an intimation of something people knew of through the influence of Zoroastrian culture; and from there awareness of Ahriman spread to other peoples and informed their cultural ideas. Ahriman and his hosts surfaced in different cultures under the most diverse names. European souls who had remained furthest behind during west-east migrations, and had therefore been least affected by what had occurred in ancient India, ancient Persia, in Egypt and even during the Graeco-Roman era, had a particular disposition. Upon these people of Europe, amongst whom the fifth cultural epoch was to flourish, the figure of Ahriman made an especially terrible impression. Elsewhere taking the most varied names—such as Mephistopheles in Hebrew culture—he became the figure of the devil in his various forms in Europe.

Thus we can gain insight into a profound reality of worlds of spirit; and on occasion, if someone feels justified in looking askance at medieval superstition, it might be good to recall what our *Faust* poet said: 'Small folk never sense the devil, even if he has them by the scruff!'[41]

Precisely by closing their eyes to this influence, people are most in thrall to it. Goethe's Mephistopheles is none other than the figure of Ahriman, and we should not confuse him with Lucifer. All the mistakes we encounter in critical analyses of Goethe's *Faust* are attributable to this confusion—although of course Lucifer was the one who first made Ahriman's influence possible. When we study Ahriman, therefore, we are led back to Lucifer's primeval influence—which we have only been able to consider after long preparatory studies necessary for gaining insight into these more intimate circumstances.

We must not overlook this subtle distinction since above all Lucifer really only subjected humankind to the influence of powers connected with forces of wind and water. By contrast, Ahriman-Mephistopheles yoked us to powers that are far, far more terrible; and in forthcoming civilizations phenomena will come to the fore that are connected with his influence. Esoteric seekers who do not base their practice on solid and safe foundations can very easily fall prey to the most dreadful illusion and deception, precisely through ahrimanic influence. Ahriman is indeed a spirit who seeks to spread deception about the true nature of the sensory world, specifically by concealing the fact that this world is an expression of the world of spirit. If someone is already predisposed to abnormal states, somnambulistic conditions or, through certain types of mistaken schooling, awakens esoteric powers in himself while retaining qualities that urge him towards self-aggrandizement and egoism, then Ahriman or Mephistopheles will easily exert an influence on such esoteric powers, and this influence can become extremely powerful. Lucifer's influence only extends to manifesting in astral form—as a form that becomes visible for the astral body—things encountered by someone, even if he is engaged in a false path of schooling, that originate in the world of spirit. By contrast, the forms attributable to Ahriman's effect manifest when harmful influences to which the physical body is exposed imprint themselves into the etheric body, and then become visible as phantoms.

In the case of Ahriman's influence, therefore, we find powers at work that are far more vile than those connected with Lucifer's influence. The influences exerted by Lucifer can never become as harmful as those of Ahriman and the entities connected with fire powers. The influence of

Ahriman or Mephistopheles can affect someone to such a degree that he is induced, let us say, to undertake measures involving his physical body in order to acquire esoteric insight. The worst means one can employ to gain access to esoteric powers involve physical measures and misuse of the body. In certain schools of black magic such measures are very extensively taught. To take the physical forces of the body as the starting point for esoteric schooling is one of the direst temptations that may seduce us.

It is not possible to examine this in more detail here, except to point out that all machinations involving any misuse of the body's physical forces originate in the influences of Ahriman. This works as a phantom because it penetrates the human ether body—but such a world of phantoms is nothing other than the guise of powers that drag human beings down below the human level. Almost all cultures—the Indian, Persian, Egyptian and Graeco-Roman—underwent a period of decadence and decline into which they fell, and into which the mysteries likewise fell when the pure mystery tradition was no longer preserved. At such times many of those who were either pupils of the initiates, yet were unable to stay at their level, or people to whom esoteric secrets were wrongfully revealed, embarked on such misguided and harmful paths. These influences inspired centres of black magic power that have survived right into our own time.

Ahriman is a spirit of lies who conjures illusions before human beings, yet who works with his accomplices in a world of spirit. He himself is not an illusion—certainly not! But the apparitions conjured before a person's eye of spirit are deceptive chimeras. If a person's wishes, passions and desires pursue the wrong path while, at the same time, he gives himself up in some way to occult forces, then the occult forces that emerge in consequence penetrate his ether body. Then the most corrupt and harmful forces appear amongst the chimeras—which can sometimes assume very noble forms. That is how dire the influence of Ahriman can be on human beings.

You can see therefore that—if we wish to put it like this—Christ's appearance laid Ahriman in chains, although only for those who increasingly attempt to grasp fully the Christ mystery. Protection against Ahriman's influence will weaken increasingly apart from the powers that stream out from the Christ mystery. In a sense our time—as many occurrences show—is heading towards these influences of Ahriman. Certain secret doctrines also call Ahriman's hosts the Asuras.[42] These of course are the evil Asuras who in a certain way lapsed from the evolutionary trajectory of the Asuras responsible for endowing humankind with personality. I have indicated already that these are spiritual beings who sundered themselves from the earth's whole evolution prior to the sun's departure.

I have only described here in a preliminary way the terrible influence that Ahriman can exert on a certain course of abnormal development possible on occult paths. But in some respects the whole of humanity placed itself under the sway of Ahriman's influence during the second half of the Atlantean period. The whole post-Atlantean period contains, in a sense, the repercussions of Ahriman's influence, more in some parts of the globe and less in others. Ahriman's influence, though, made itself felt everywhere; and everything in the ancient teachings of initiates to their peoples was given by the spirits of light opposed to Ahriman, and was basically intended to enable human beings to withdraw gradually from Ahriman's influence. This was a preparatory, well-governed and wise education of humanity.

Let us not forget however that since that time Ahriman's destiny is, really, interwoven with that of humanity in a certain way, and that the most diverse occurrences of which the uninitiated can know nothing maintain a continuous connection between the karma of humanity and that of Ahriman. To understand what I am about to say, we have to be clear that besides our own individual karma general karmic laws apply at all levels of existence. All types of being have their karma, varying from one to the other. But karma itself imbues all realms of existence, and there are certainly things in humanity's karma, in the karma of a race or nation, of a society or any other human group, which we must regard as a common or shared karma. In other words, under certain circumstances the individual can be drawn into general karma. And for those who do not fully comprehend these things it is not always easy to recognize the source of the powers that inflict this fate on people. An individual embedded in a larger social context may be quite innocent as far as his individual karma is concerned, but can suffer misfortune because he participates in the overall karma. If he is truly innocent, though, this will be compensated and redressed in subsequent incarnations.

In extending our view of these things we should not consider past karma only, but also future karma. It is certainly true to say that under certain circumstances there can be a whole social group that suffers a terrible fate, and it can be hard to discover why this fate was inflicted on that group. Someone in a position to study individual karma may not be able to discover anything at all that might have led to this sad destiny, for karmic connections are very intricate and convoluted. What requires such karma to manifest in one way or another may have very, very distant—yet still connected—causes. A whole, innocent group may also suffer a general karma whereas those directly at fault could be left unscathed due to the lack of any opportunity for karma to act. In such cases, all we can say is this: in the general karma of an individual everything is balanced and redressed even if he is innocently struck down in one way or another. It is inscribed in his karma, and at some point in the future will be fully redressed. Thus in studying the law of karma, we must also consider future karma. But we should not forget either that an individual is not a separate, isolated being. Every individual must share in bearing the common karma of humanity. Nor should we forget that as human beings and thus part of humanity we belong at the same time to the hierarchies of beings who have not entered the physical world, and that we are also involved in the karma of these hierarchies. Aspects of fate and destiny in the physical world can be embedded in a context that has no immediate connection with directly related things, although karmic consequences inevitably arise. Since the second half of the Atlantean period, Ahriman's karma has been connected with that of humanity. Besides his effect on physical human bodies to instil illusion and phantoms in us about the sensory world, where else should we seek the deeds of Ahriman? Where else can we discover them?

We can say that there are two sides to everything in the world: one that belongs more to the human being as a spiritual being, and another that belongs to what has formed and developed around us as the kingdoms of nature. The earth is the human being's stage and arena.

The eye of spirit finds the earth to be an interrelated whole containing diverse layers. We know that the outermost layer of our earth is called the mineral earth or mineral layer since it contains only the substances that we find beneath our feet. This is relatively speaking the thinnest stratum. Then begins the pliant earth, which has a quite different material structure from the mineral layer above it. You can say that this second stratum is endowed with inner life. The inner forces of this second layer are only held together because the solid, mineral layer spreads over it. If they were ever released, these forces would disperse throughout the heavens. Thus this layer is under an enormous pressure. The vapour layer is the third. This is not vapour of a material kind, though, as we are familiar with on the earth's surface, but here, in the third layer, substance itself is endowed with inner forces we can only compare with human passions, with inner drives. Whereas above on the earth only beings constituted as animals and humans can develop drives and passions, this third layer is materially permeated—in the very same way that the earth's substances are permeated by forces of magnetism and heat—by forces identical to what we know as human and animal drives and passions. The fourth layer is the layer of forms, so named because it contains the material and forces of what we encounter in the earth's mineral realm as formed entities. And the fifth layer, the fruit earth, is distinguished by the infinite fertility of its own intrinsic material. If you had a part of this layer of the earth, it would continually sprout new shoots and scions from itself. The element of this layer is burgeoning fertility. After this we come to the sixth layer, the fire earth, containing substances that can act in terribly devastating and destructive ways. These forces are the ones, really, into which primal fires have been banished.

It is in this layer, basically, that the realm of Ahriman holds material sway, and its activity stems from there. What appears in external natural phenomena in air and water, in cloud formations, in thunder and lightning is, you can say, a last vestige on the earth's surface—but a good one—of forces already connected with Old Saturn, which departed with the sun. Drawn from what works in these forces, the earth's inner fire forces serve Ahriman, and here he has the centre of his actions. Whereas his spiritual effects enter human souls in the way described, leading them into error, we see how—chained in a certain way—he has focus points of influence in the earth's interior. If people understood the mysterious connections between what has occurred on earth under Ahriman's influence and what has become Ahriman's own karma in consequence, they would recognize in earth eruptions, in earthquakes, the relationship between such tragic, appalling natural events and what holds sway on the earth. This has remained over from ancient times as something that reacts on earth against light-filled, benevolent beings.

All over the earth, then, work forces of one kind or another connected with beings that were repulsed from the earth at the time when light-filled, benevolent beings governed wholesome, beneficial phenomena at work around the globe. In a sense we can recognize the echo of these fire effects, withdrawn from human beings in former times, in the harm done by fire in such appalling natural phenomena. There is no need to think that people who suffer such events, caused by Ahriman's karma—which has however been connected with humanity's karma since Atlantean times—are in any way at fault. Such things are connected with the whole karma of humanity, in which each individual also has a share. The results of Ahriman's karma, coming to effect in certain places, are often attributable to causes that lie elsewhere entirely. It is just that such places offer an opportunity for these effects to manifest.

Here we see a context that can appear to us, however, as a residual throwback to other primeval catastrophes that affected humanity. In Lemurian times, human beings were deprived of the power of acting upon fire. Previously they had the capacity to do so. Ancient Lemuria perished as a result of the fire passions of humankind. The fire that is now in the earth's interior was then upon its surface, and withdrew into the depths. The same fire that emerged as an extract of the primeval fire exists today as our inorganic, mineral fire. The same thing occurred with the forces active in air and water which, due to human passions, caused the Atlantean catastrophes. These catastrophes were invoked by the karma of all humanity; but a residue remained and this calls forth echoes of these catastrophes. Our volcanic eruptions and earthquakes are nothing other than the echoes or reverberations of these catastrophes. But it is important to remember that it would be quite wrong

to attribute any blame whatever to someone affected by such a catastrophe, or that compassion should be withheld from those affected. An
anthroposophist must be clear that the karma of such people has no
bearing on his own actions towards them, and that he must not
withhold help because—in a trivial sense—he believes in karma and
therefore thinks a person brought this fate upon himself. Karma in fact
calls on us to help others, since we can be certain that our help signifies
something for them that will be inscribed in their karma and guide it in
a more favourable direction.

An understanding of the world founded on karma must lead to
compassion. Such understanding will render us all the more com-
passionate towards misfortunate people who suffer such catastrophes.
For it tells us that individual members of humanity have to bear the
consequences of humanity's overall karma, and that just as the whole of
humanity brings about such occurrences the whole of humanity likewise
must take responsibility for each of us acknowledging this destiny as our
own. It is not even a voluntary act of good will to help others, but such
action must be based on knowing that we are fully implicated in the
karma of humanity, and that we too owe whatever debt is owing.

I was sent a question this morning that relates to earthquake catastrophes. It was this:

> *What is the esoteric explanation of earthquake catastrophes? Can they be*
> *predicted? If such catastrophes could be predicted in advance, would it not*
> *be possible to issue some kind of quiet warning? Such a warning might not*
> *be much use the first time, but later people would doubtless take notice of it.*

Our older members will recall what was said, at the end of the lecture
on 'The Interior of the Earth',[43] about possible factors relating to
earthquakes. But we will pass over that now and deal directly with this
question. It has two parts, really: firstly, whether earthquakes might be
predicted through insight into their esoteric context. The answer is this:
understanding of such matters belongs to the most profound esoteric
knowledge. A single such event that occurs on the earth, originating
largely in profound causes such as have been described today, is connected with factors that go far beyond the earth itself. In such an
instance, it is basically absolutely correct to say that it can be predicted

for a specific time. The seer would certainly be able to predict this. But the other question is this: Can we, or ought we to issue such warnings? For anyone who takes an exoteric view of esoteric secrets, it will appear almost self-evident that the answer could be 'yes' in certain circumstances. Yet in fact, in relation to such events, initiation centres could issue such predictions no more than two or three times each century—two or three times at the very most. You see, you must remember that these things are connected with humanity's karma, and even if they could be avoided in individual instances, they would have to surface again in another form. This fact could not be altered by advance prediction. Consider too what a terrible intervention in the karma of the whole earth it would be if human measures could be taken to avoid such events! It would elicit an appalling reaction, so powerful in nature that only in rare and exceptional cases could a high initiate, aware of a forthcoming earthquake, make use of his knowledge for himself or for those closest to him. Despite his knowledge he would simply have to forfeit his life. You see, these things that lie in the karma of humanity through thousands and millions of years cannot be halted by relatively short-term measures that fall within a brief period of human destiny. But another factor must be considered as well.

We have seen that this domain belongs to the most difficult areas of esoteric research. When I gave my lecture on the earth's interior, I said how enormously difficult it is to know anything about this interior; and that it is far easier to know about astral space, devachan and even the furthest planets than about the earth's interior. Most things said about the interior of the earth are complete drivel, since this realm is one of the hardest esoteric domains to understand. It is one that also includes things connected with these elemental catastrophes. Above all you must keep in mind that clairvoyance is not something which involves just sitting down, invoking a particular state and then being able to say what is happening everywhere in the world, through to its loftiest realms. This is not so. Such thinking is as perceptive as saying to someone: 'You can see things in the physical world, so why didn't you see what was going on at noon by the river while you were sitting here in the room?' There are hindrances to vision. If the person in question had gone for a walk at noon, he might well have seen what happened. It is not true to say that simply by putting oneself in the right state of awareness one can immediately perceive all worlds at the same time. Here too a person has to first go towards whatever he wishes to study, and examine it; and the investigations involved in this case are among the most difficult of all, since the greatest hindrances obstruct vision. It may perhaps be appropriate to speak about such hindrances here.

You can deprive a person of the capacity to walk physically on two legs not only by cutting off his legs but also by locking him up, thus preventing him from walking about. Likewise there are hindrances to esoteric enquiries, and in the realm we are speaking of there are indeed huge obstacles. I would like to describe one of the chief hindrances now, pointing you towards mysterious circumstances. The biggest obstacle to esoteric research in this domain is the way in which external, materialistic science is practised nowadays. The endless illusions and errors that accumulate in materialistic science, all the undignified research that is undertaken, not only leading to no outcome but really only proceeding from human vanity, are things whose effects in higher worlds render research about the phenomena we have been discussing impossible in these higher worlds, curtailing a free view or at least greatly hampering it. An open vista there is obscured due to the materialistic research undertaken here on earth.

These things are not straightforward or easy to survey. I'll put it like this. Let us await a time when spiritual science becomes more widespread so that, through its influence, materialistic superstitions about our world are swept away! Random combining and setting up of hypotheses projects every possible fantasy into the earth's interior, but once all this has been swept away you will see how spiritual science at last comes to integrate itself into the karma of humanity. It will find the ways and means to engage souls and by virtue of this will be able to conquer adversary powers and materialistic superstition, investigating further all that is connected with the worst enemy of humanity, who chains the human gaze to the sensory world. You will then see that this also opens up the possibility of acting outwardly on human karma by assuaging the terrible nature of such events. Examine the materialistic superstitions of human beings to discover why initiates must remain silent about events connected with the great karma of humanity.

Science is mostly not informed by a Faustian striving for truth but instead is completely pervaded by vanity and ambition. So much scientific research that makes headway in the world arises from an individual's own self-seeking. If you add this all up, you will see how strong is the power that unfolds to obscure a vista of the world concealed behind external sensory phenomena. Once humanity has swept this fog away, the time will arrive when it is possible to offer extensive help to diminish the effects of certain mysterious natural phenomena emanating from humanity's enemies and impacting strongly on human life. Until then, this will not be possible.

I do realize that the questioner did not necessarily expect his question to take us where it has. But in some matters, you see, esoteric doctrine is destined first to redirect a question so that it can be properly formulated, before it can be answered correctly. But do not take this to mean, either, that the mysterious connection between earth catastrophes and humanity's karma is one of the secrets that cannot be studied or investigated. It can be. Yet there are reasons why only very general aspects of these most profound secrets can find their way into the world. Once humanity has come to discern, through spiritual science, the possibility of a connection between human deeds and natural events, then, precisely through this insight, the time will also arrive when humanity comes to see how such questions can receive an appropriate reply. This time will come, for spiritual science can pass through various destinies of its own. Its influence may even come to a standstill, restricted to the narrowest circles. But it will nevertheless make its way through humanity and find its way into the karma of humanity. And then it will become possible for humanity itself to act upon and influence its own karma.

Lecture 13

During this winter, as I have stated already in these sessions, the aim is to compile the materials, the different building blocks of each lecture, so that together they eventually offer deeper insight into the nature of the human being and various other things connected with human life and evolution, thus leading us ever deeper into secrets of the universe. Today I want to recall the lecture before last[44] as our point of departure. You will remember that we spoke about a certain rhythm that exists in relation to the four aspects or levels of the human being. That is where we will begin today, trying to answer this question: How can such knowledge, drawing on deeper foundations, give us insight into the need for and aim of the anthroposophical spiritual movement?

We will need to link two apparently very divergent things today. You recall that certain relationships exist between the human I, astral body, ether body and physical body. What can be said of the fourth level, the I, appears, one might say, in the most tangible form to us if we think of the two alternating states of consciousness which the I undergoes during the 24-hour period of a day. This single day with its 24 hours, during which the I experiences day and night, sleeping and waking, can in a sense be regarded as one unit. If we say that what the I experiences during a single day is subject to the number one, then the number corresponding in similar fashion to our astral body is seven. While we can say that the I, as it is today, returns to its starting point after 24 hours, or one day, our astral body does the same in seven days. Let us examine this in somewhat more detail.

Think of waking up in the morning, which involves what people commonly regard—though of course wrongly—as surfacing from the darkness of unconsciousness so that the objects of the physical, sensory world reappear around you. You experience this in the morning and usually at least have the same experience again 24 hours later. That is what usually happens, and we can say that our I returns to its starting point after one day of 24 hours. In the same way, we can seek corresponding relationships for the astral body and will find that where the regularity proper to the human astral body actually manifests it returns to the same point again after seven days. Whereas the I passes through a one-day cycle, the astral body goes a good deal more slowly, passing through its cycle in seven days. The ether body passes through its cycle in four times seven days, returning to the same point again after this period. And now I would ask you to note what I said in the lecture before last: there is not the same regularity for the physical body as for the astral and ether body, but we can establish an approximate cycle of roughly ten times 28 days, after which it returns to its starting point. You know of course that there is an important distinction to be made in that the human female ether body is male in character while the male ether body is female. This can show us that in certain respects there is an inevitable irregularity between the ether body rhythm and that of the physical body. But generally speaking the ratios between the four levels of human nature—what we can call their 'speed of rotation'—are: $1:7:(4 \times 7):(10 \times 7 \times 4)$. Naturally this is only a metaphor, for rotations do not occur as such but cyclical repetitions of the same states. These are rhythmic ratios. A fortnight ago[45] I indicated that occurrences in our daily life can only be understood if we know that such things underlie the physical world of the senses. And in a public lecture,[46] too, I pointed to a remarkable fact which even the most materialistic of researchers and physicians cannot deny, since it exists as a reality and cannot be classified as a 'phantom of superstition'. This is the fact—which ought really to give people pause for thought—that a crisis occurs seven days after pneumonia begins, which the patient must be helped to survive. Fever suddenly drops, and if one does not help the patient over this crisis he may not recover. This fact is commonly acknowledged, but the starting date of the illness is not always correctly ascertained; and if one does not know what day the disease began, it is easy to be unaware of its seventh day. This is a fact nevertheless. And so we must ask why fever drops on the seventh day of pneumonia. Why does something specific happen on day seven?

Only someone who can look behind the veils of existence, seeing into the world of spirit underlying physical phenomena, knows of these rhythms and at the same time understands what gives rise to phenomena such as fever. What is fever really? Why does it arise? Fever is not disease but, on the contrary, something the organism invokes to combat the actual process of disease. It is the organism's defence against disease when there is some deficiency or damage in the organism, say in the lungs. When we are healthy, and all our internal functions are in harmony, these internal functions will inevitably be disturbed if an organ, any part of the human body, suffers a disorder. In this case the whole organism will try to mobilize, drawing from itself the forces to remedy this specific disorder. A revolution occurs in the whole organism. When no enemy is present to be combated, the organism has no need to muster its forces. Fever is the expression of this mustering of forces in the organism.

Someone who can look behind the veils of existence knows that the germ of different human organs was laid down, and developed, at very different periods of human evolution. Spiritual-scientific 'study of the human body', as we may call it, is the most complex imaginable field, since this human organism is very diverse and its various organs originated at very different times. The original germ was later taken up again and developed further. Everything in the human organism is an expression, an outcome, of the human being's higher aspects, such that any part of the physical body expresses the laws of higher levels. The lungs, as we refer to them today, are originally intrinsically connected with the human astral body, and have something to do with it. We will return to the subject of how the lungs are connected with the astral body, how the very first, primal beginnings of the lungs were incorporated into the human being at the planetary stage preceding our earth, that of old Moon, and how higher spiritual beings as it were 'instilled' the astral body in us. Today we will just note that the lungs are, among much else, an expression of the astral body. The true expression of the astral body is of course the nervous system. But the human being is complex, and evolutionary processes always run parallel to each other. The incipient lungs arose along with the evolution of the astral body and incorporation of today's nervous system. Because of this, the lungs engage in a certain way in the astral body's rhythm—which is subject to a periodicity governed by the number seven. Symptoms of fever are connected with certain functions of the ether body. Something has to happen in the ether body for fever to take its course. Fever therefore stands somehow within the same rhythm as the ether body. Every fever is involved in this rhythm, but how? We must now clarify the following.

Since the ether body accomplishes its cycle in four times seven days, it moves a good deal more slowly than the astral body, whose cycle lasts seven days. If we relate the rhythmic periodicity of the ether body to that of the astral body, we can compare this with the hands of a clock. The hour hand goes once around the clock-face while the minute hand completes twelve circuits during the same period, giving the ratio of 1:12. Now imagine glancing at the clock at midday when the hour hand stands directly over the minute hand so that the two are super-imposed. Then the minute hand continues to move, completing one more circuit. Returning to the 12 it will no longer cover the hour hand since the latter has moved to the 1, and the two hands will then only coincide again after around five minutes. In other words, the minute hand will not cover the hour hand again after an hour but after an hour and a little over five minutes. The relationship between the cycle of the astral body and that of the ether body is similar to this. Let us assume that your astral body—which is of course always linked with the ether body—is in a certain condition in relation to the latter. Now the astral body starts to rotate. After seven days, when it returns to its original condition, it no longer coincides with the ether body, for the latter has by then advanced through a quarter of its own cycle. At the end of seven days, therefore, the condition of the astral body no longer coincides with the same condition of the ether body but instead with a condition that lags behind the original one by a quarter of the cycle. Now assume that the disease in question develops. Here a quite specific condition of the astral body is connected with a quite specific condition of the ether body. At this moment, fever arises with the participation of these two concurrent conditions, as a mustering of forces to combat the enemy. After seven days the astral body coincides with a quite different point of the ether body. The ether body requires more than the strength to produce fever, for otherwise, once it had got the fever going, this fever would never cease. After seven days, the point of the ether body, which now coincides with the point of the astral body that engendered fever seven days before, has the tendency to remedy the fever—to assuage and diminish it. If, after seven days, the patient has overcome the disorder, things will go well. But if not, and if the astral body now has no inclination to fight off the illness, it will encounter an unfavourable condition where the ether body tends to diminish the fever. We must take careful note of these two superimposed points, these points of coincidence—and we could establish their presence in all kinds of factors relating to human life. Precisely through these rhythms, through mysterious inner mechanisms, the whole nature of the human being could become clear to us. The ether body does indeed tend to express itself in a cycle of four times seven. In other illnesses, in turn, you can observe the special importance of the fourteenth day, thus twice seven. In certain conditions we can demonstrate that paroxysm will be particularly pronounced after four times seven days. And in this case, if the severity of the disease abates, there can be sure hope of recovery. All these things are connected with rhythms, notably the ones we touched on three weeks ago, which we have now examined in more detail. Such matters, seemingly difficult but understandable nevertheless, allow us to delve a little behind the surface of the physical world of the senses. And we must delve ever deeper. Now let us ask about the specific origins of such rhythms.

These rhythms originate in great cosmic relationships. We have repeatedly described the past evolution through Saturn, Sun, Moon and Earth stages of what we call the four bodies or aspects of the human being—physical body, ether body, astral body and I. If we look back to the old Moon embodiment, we discover that this too separated from the sun for a certain period. At that time, however, a great part of what is today's moon was connected with the earth. A sun stood separate from it, though, and when such heavenly bodies belong together, their forces—which are in turn only an expression of their living entities—always exert an influence on the regularity of the life of their indwelling entities. The time a planet takes to orbit the sun, or that a satellite takes to orbit its planet, is certainly not accidental or unconnected with living realities, but is governed by beings we have come to know in the hierarchies of spirits. We have learned, indeed, that the orbits of heavenly bodies are not caused by mere soulless forces. On one occasion we described the grotesque fashion in which a modern physicist demonstrates the Kant-Laplace theory by means of a floating drop of fat. A cardboard disc is inserted through the drop of fat in line with the equator, while a needle pierces it from above; and now the whole thing is rotated—whereupon small drops split off from the large one and are drawn into the same rotational movement. Thus an experimenter shows how a planetary system arises on a small scale, and from this in general the physicist concludes how our solar system must have arisen. The factor it is otherwise a good idea to forget—oneself—is a stumbling block in this instance. For you see, the good fellow will usually overlook the fact that the little planetary system could not form without him cranking the engine. Of course such experiments can be done, and are very useful, but in doing them we ought not to forget the vital factor. Countless people mistakenly absorb such suggestions, forgetting that their esteemed professor himself was the *primum mobile*. There is no giant professor out in the universe, it is true, but his place is taken by the hierarchies of spiritual beings who govern the heavenly bodies' motions and cycles. They do indeed configure cosmic matter so that individual planets orbit one another. And if—as will be possible some day—we could study in more detail the movements of the planets, which constitute a unified system, we would rediscover in them the rhythms of our own supersensible bodies. Initially, though, we need only highlight one thing.

Materialistic ways of thinking mean that people today laugh at how, in former times, certain human circumstances were linked with the moon's quarters. But in a wonderful fashion the moon cosmically reflects a relationship between the astral body and the ether body. The moon passes through its cycle in four times seven days. These are the conditions of the ether body, and the four times seven ether body conditions are fully reflected in the moon's four quarters. It is far from nonsense to seek in the moon's quarters a connection with the fever symptoms we described above. After seven days, a new quarter is present, you see, like a new quarter of the ether body, so that the astral body coincides with a different quarter of the ether body. This relationship of human astral and ether bodies was in fact originally governed by the fact that spiritual beings caused the moon to orbit the earth in a corresponding way. You can gather that these things are connected from the fact that even modern medicine draws on an old vestige of rhythmic insight. It is because the rhythm of the physical body consists of 10×28, so that after 10×28 days the physical body returns, as it were, to the point it occupied previously, that there is a period of roughly 10×28 days between human conception and birth— ten sidereal months. All these things are connected with the way great cosmic relationships are regulated. The human being is a microcosm that faithfully reflects great universal relationships, and is constituted by them.

Today we will consider the evolutionary period that falls in the middle of Atlantean times, a very important point in earth's evolution. In humanity's evolution we distinguish three previous races: the first the Polaric, the second the Hyperborean and the third the Lemurian race. We are now in the fifth race, which will be followed by two further ones, and the Atlantean period lies at the midpoint of evolution. The middle of Atlantean times is the most important point of earth's evolution. If we were to go back before this time we would find that the outward conditions of human life exactly reflect cosmic conditions. In those times things would have gone very badly for human beings if they had done what they do today. Today people no longer orientate themselves much in accordance with cosmic conditions. In our cities, of course, circumstances are such that a person will stay awake when he ought to sleep and sleep when he ought to be awake. If anything similar to staying awake at night and sleeping during the day had occurred in Lemurian times, and if people had paid such little attention to how outer phenomena correspond with inner processes, they would have been unable to live at all. Such a thing, of course, would have been impossible, since in those times it was entirely self-evident that people's inner rhythm was governed by an external rhythm. In those days people lived in harmony with the course of the sun and moon, precisely attuning to these the rhythm of their astral body and ether body.

Let us take a clock once more. In a sense a clock too is oriented to the great course of the heavens. Whenever the hour hand coincides with the minute hand at 12 o'clock, this is because a particular solar and sidereal constellation exists. The clock is governed by this, and runs badly if, a day later, it does not bring these two hands together when this same sidereal constellation occurs. From the observatory at Enckeplatz, electrical connections daily regulate the clocks in Berlin. So we can say that these movements, these rhythms, correspond to the clock-hands, which are even coordinated with them on a daily basis. Our clock runs accurately when it corresponds to the master clock which, in turn, accords with the cosmos. In ancient times, in fact, people did not need clocks for they themselves were clocks. They regulated the course of their lives, of which they had a very tangible sense, according to cosmic conditions and relationships. The human being really was a clock. And if he had not oriented himself to cosmic conditions then exactly the same would have happened to him as happens with a clock if it is at odds with outer reality: it runs badly; and human beings would then also have been in a bad way. The inner rhythm had to accord with the outer.

A major aspect of human progress on earth is that, since the middle of Atlantean times, outer and inner circumstances have no longer been in absolute accord. Something else has arisen. Imagine if someone had the quirk of not wanting the two hands of his clock to coincide at 12 o'clock. Let's assume he set his clock so that it showed 3 o'clock at that moment. His clock would show 4 p.m. when it was 1 p.m. for everyone else, and 5 p.m. when it was 2 p.m. But this would not alter the workings of his clock: it would just be out of sequence with outer circumstances. After 24 hours his clock will show 3 o'clock again, and will therefore be out of sync with cosmic relationships. In its own internal rhythm, though, it will accord with them, simply transposing or shifting it. In the same way, the human being's rhythm was transposed, and we would never have become autonomous beings if our whole activity had been tied to the apron strings of cosmic conditions. We acquired freedom precisely by releasing ourselves from the external rhythm while nevertheless retaining the same inner rhythm. We became like a clock that no longer coincides with cosmic events at key junctures, yet still inwardly accords with them. In ancient times of the primeval past a human being could only be conceived at a very specific zodiac constellation, and was then born ten lunar months later. This concurrence of conception with a cosmic condition fell away, but the rhythm itself remained, just as the rhythm of a clock is retained even if one sets it to 3 o'clock at midday. However, besides our own condition, periodicity itself also shifted. But if we ignore this cosmic shift, something very particular happened to the human being by virtue of the fact that he detached himself from cosmic circumstances, and is therefore no longer a 'clock' in the true sense of the word. What occurred for him is what would happen to someone who sets his clock fast by three hours, but then forgets how much he has advanced it, and therefore no longer knows how things stand. The same happened to us during earth evolution once we departed from our clocklike relationship with the cosmos. In certain respects we caused disorder in our astral body. The more the circumstances of human life correlated with corporeal reality, the more the ancient rhythm was retained; but as circumstances adapted increasingly to spiritual reality, the greater was the disorder into which they fell. I would like to explain this from another perspective as well.

Besides human beings we know of beings at a higher level than humanity on earth today. We know of the sons of life, or angels, who passed through their 'humanity stage' on old Moon. We know the fire spirits or archangels who underwent stages of human evolution on the earth's old Sun embodiment, and likewise we know the primal powers who passed through their humanity stage on old Saturn. In cosmic evolution, these beings ran ahead of human beings. If we studied them today we would find that they are far more spiritual in nature than the human being, and therefore also live in higher worlds. But in relation to what we have spoken of today they find themselves in a quite different position from us. They orient themselves spiritually in full accord with the rhythm of the cosmos. An angel would never think in such a disordered way as a human being, simply because his trains of thought are governed by the cosmic powers which orient him. It is simply inconceivable for a being such as an angel to think in any other way than in harmony with great spiritual, cosmic processes. The laws of angelic logic are inscribed in the universal harmony. They have no need of text-books—whereas we do because we have brought disorder into our inner modes of thinking. People no longer perceive how to orient themselves in accordance with the great sidereal script. These angels know how the cosmos unfolds, and their trains of thinking correspond to a regulated rhythm. When the human being began to walk on earth in his current form, he detached himself from this rhythm, and thus his thinking, feelings and emotions are random. Whereas regularity prevails in things we have less influence over—the astral and ether body—irregularity and arrhythmia, lack of rhythm have entered the aspects we ourselves have taken in hand, namely our sentient soul, mind soul and con-sciousness soul. The least of this is apparent in the way we turn night into day in big cities. What is far more significant is that people have sundered themselves from the great universal rhythms in their mode of thinking. The way they think at every moment in some respects con-tradicts the great motions of the spheres.

Now please don't imagine that I have said all this to propound a world-view that seeks to reintegrate human beings into a rhythm of this kind. We had to emerge from the ancient rhythm of existence, and progress depends on this. When 'back-to-nature' prophets preach today, they want to push life back to where it started rather than advance it. Dabbling like this in vague ideas about going back to nature shows a failure to understand evolution. A movement urging people today to eat certain foods only at certain seasons, since nature itself indicates this by growing particular foods at specific times of year, represents a completely abstract kind of amateurism. Evolution consists precisely in increasing human independence from an external rhythm. But we should not lose the ground under our feet either. Our true, salutary progress is not furthered by returning to the old rhythm of life—asking, say, how one can live in harmony with the four quarters of the moon. This is a throwback to ancient times when it was necessary for us to be a kind of seal or imprint of the cosmos. On the other hand, though, it is also important not to think that we can live without rhythm. In the same way that we became internalized from without, we must now reconfigure ourselves rhythmically from within. This is the important thing. Rhythm must imbue our inner life.

As rhythm developed the cosmos so must we—if we wish to participate in the development of a new cosmos—permeate ourselves with new rhythm. It is characteristic of our age that it has lost the old rhythm without as yet developing a new one. As human beings we have outgrown nature—if we regard nature as the outward manifestation of spirit—without so far growing back into spirit. We are still dangling somewhere between nature and spirit, and this characterizes our age. This floundering about between nature and spirit reached its culmination in the second third of the nineteenth century. This was why the beings who recognize and interpret the signs of the times asked what needed to be done to prevent human beings losing rhythm altogether, and allow an inner rhythm to penetrate them once again.

Disorder and irregularity characterize modern culture. Whenever you see a cultural artefact of any kind the first thing that will strike you about it is its disorderly, inwardly irregular nature. This is true in almost all areas. Only disciplines still based on solid old traditions still retain something of their old regularity. In new fields we still need to create a new regularity. This is why, despite ascertaining facts such as the drop of temperature in a pneumonia patient on day seven of the disease, the reasons thought up to explain this are simply chaotic. When someone thinks about such things, instead of thinking in a regular, ordered way he piles a whole mish-mash of thoughts on top of one other. In all scientific disciplines researchers take a verifiable fact and then stir up a pile of thoughts about it, without any inner regularity. People today have no inner lines of thought or rhythm of thinking; and humanity would lapse into complete decadence if it did not, in fact, absorb an inner rhythm. Take a look at spiritual science from this perspective for a moment.

You can see what sort of waters you enter when you start engaging with spiritual science. First you hear—and gradually come to understand—that the human being consists of four aspects: physical body, ether body, astral body and I. And then you hear how the I acts upon the others, transforming the astral body into Manas or Spirit Self, transforming the ether body into Buddhi or Life Spirit and transforming our physical principle, the physical body, into Spirit Man or Atma. Now just consider for a moment how this basic formula, as it were, of our spiritual science informs so much of what we study. Think of the many themes, basic themes really, that were built up repeatedly in our overall edifice of thoughts from an initial schema of physical body, ether body, astral body and I. As you know, some people even grow weary of hearing these fundamental facts repeatedly reiterated at public lectures. But it is and remains a sure thread through our developing sequences of thought: these four aspects of human nature, the way they work together, and then in turn the higher transformation of the lower three levels—of the third into the fifth, the second into the sixth and the first into the seventh aspect of our being. If you now take all of them together there are seven: physical body, ether body, astral body, I, Spirit Self, Life Spirit and Spirit Man. And taking what underlies them— physical body, ether body, astral body and I—there are four. Thus, in considering these sequences you repeat in your thoughts the great rhythm of 7:4, or 4:7. You reproduce from within you this great external rhythm, repeating the rhythm that once existed on a large scale in the universal cosmos—you give birth to it again. In doing so you are laying down the plan, the foundation, for your thought system in the same way that the gods once laid down the plan for the world's wisdom. In this way a cosmos of thought evolves within the soul when we revive within us the inner rhythm of number as I have just outlined. Human beings have emancipated themselves from external rhythm. Through a spiritual science worthy of the name we return to rhythm, building from within outwards a world edifice that bears rhythm within it. And if we pass on to the cosmos and consider the earth's past forms, studying Saturn, Sun, Moon and Earth, we find a fourfold sequence in which the old Moon stage returns in spiritualized form at the fifth stage as Jupiter, old Sun returns at the sixth stage as Venus, and old Saturn reappears at the seventh stage as Vulcan. Thus in Saturn, Sun, Moon, Earth, Jupiter, Venus and Vulcan we have our sevenfold evolutionary phases. Our physical body as it is today, evolved through the four stages, through Saturn, Sun, Moon and Earth. In future it will gradually be wholly reconfigured and spiritualized. So here too, if we look back into the past we have the number four, and the number three as we look towards the future, thus 4:3 or, if we include the past in the whole sequence of evolution, 4:7.

Though we have been preoccupied with our spiritual-scientific work and activity for many years now, we are really still only at the beginning of it. For only the first time, today, we drew attention to what people sought when they pointed to the 'inner number' upon which all phenomena are founded. Thus we see how the human being had to emerge from the original rhythm in order to secure his freedom. But we must find within ourselves again the laws whereby we regulate the 'clock', our astral body. And spiritual science is this great regulator, since it is in harmony with the great laws of the cosmos that the seer perceives. The future, as human beings create it, will show the same great numerical relationships as in the cosmos's past, but at a higher level. This is why human beings will give birth to the future out of themselves, out of number, just as the gods once formed the cosmos out of number.

And in this way we see how spiritual science is connected with the great course of the universe. When we realize what underlies us in the world of spirit as fourfold and sevenfold number, we can grasp why we must also find in this world of spirit the impulse to develop further humanity's whole previous evolutionary trajectory. And we can understand why, precisely in an age when human beings' thinking, feeling and will life have become extremely inwardly chaotic, the individualities tasked with interpreting the signs of the times have pointed to a wisdom that enables us to develop our life of soul in a regulated way, so that new rhythm emerges within us. We learn to think rhythmically, as is necessary for the future, when we think in a way that is informed by these fundamental relationships. And human beings will absorb and integrate ever more of what they are born from. Initially they extract what they must regard as the blueprint of the cosmos. Then they advance further, feeling themselves imbued by certain fundamental powers and forces, and ultimately by originating beings.

All of this stands at an initial point of departure today. And we experience the importance and world significance of the anthroposophical mission if, rather than regarding it as an arbitrary act of this or that individual, as some isolated factor, we make efforts to grasp it through the whole inner workings and impetus of our being. Then we can reach the point of saying that it is not simply up to us to accept or reject this anthroposophical mission but that, if we wish to understand our times, we must perceive and permeate ourselves with thoughts of the divine world of spirit upon which anthroposophy is founded. And in turn we must then allow this to flow out into the world so that our actions and existence develop not into a chaos but into a cosmos, in the same way that we were originally born from a cosmos.

LECTURE 14

BERLIN, 26 JANUARY 1909

LET us continue with our observations, whose aim is to enable us to understand the real nature of the human being and his task in the world from an ever deepening perspective. You will recall that in one of the lectures given here this winter[47] I spoke of the four primary ways in which human disease can manifest, saying that we would only later come to discuss what we can call the real karmic causes of disease. Today we will consider, to some extent at least, this karmic causation of disease.

On that previous occasion, describing the human being in terms of four aspects, physical body, ether body, astral body and I, we simultaneously offered a certain overview of diseases such that each of these aspects of the human being comes to expression in particular organs and organ systems of the physical body itself. Thus the I within the physical body comes largely to expression in the blood, the astral body in the nervous system, and the ether body in all that we regard as the glandular system, and what belongs to this. The physical body expresses itself as itself—as physical body. We then presented the diseases that originate in the I as such, and which therefore come to outward physical manifestation as irregularities of blood functions. We indicated that conditions caused by astral body irregularities express themselves as irregularities of the nervous system, while causes originating in the ether body express themselves in the glandular system. Then we saw how diseases we must regard as originating in the physical body are caused primarily by external factors. In all this, though, we only considered disease in relation to everything that occurs in a single life between birth and death. But someone able to draw on spiritual science when considering what unfolds in the universe will have a sense that the illnesses a person suffers must be connected in some way with his karma—that is, with the great law of causation involving spiritual connections between different incarnations. Yet the ways of karma are very convoluted, very diverse, and if we wish to understand anything at all about karmic causes and contexts, we will have to enter fully into these subtle interrelationships.

Today we will discuss a little of what people initially find it most interesting to know—how diseases are connected with causes which a person himself initiated in former lives. But to do so, by way of introduction, we must first say a few words about the workings of karma within human biography. We will need to mention some things that most of you already know from other lectures, since it is important to remind ourselves very clearly how karmic causes become effects working over from one life into another. Here we must again recall, in a few words, what happens to us during the period following death.

We know that on passing through the gate of death, the experiences we initially have are due to our being for the first time in a position we were not in during our lifetime. We have no physical body, but our I and astral body are still connected with the ether body. We have laid aside our physical body. During life this only occurs in exceptional instances, as has often been mentioned. During life, in sleep, when we lay aside the physical body, the ether body is also laid aside with it; and so this connection of I, astral body and ether body is only present for a while after death, and only for a few days. We have also spoken of the experiences during this time that follow immediately after death, describing how we feel ourselves becoming ever larger as though growing beyond the spatial bounds we previously occupied, and encompassing all things. We spoke of how the image of our past life stands before us in a great panorama. Then a period follows, varying individually and taking a matter of days in our time reckoning: the laying aside of the second corpse, the ether body, which is then absorbed into the universal ether. The only exceptions to this are the instances we have referred to when discussing delicate, intimate questions of

reincarnation, when the ether body is in a sense preserved for subsequent use. But an essence remains of this ether body, as the fruit of
what we experienced and underwent during our life. We live on after
death in this life governed by the coexistence of the I with the astral
body, now without any connection to the physical body. The time
follows which we have become accustomed to calling kamaloca in
spiritual-scientific literature, and have also often referred to as the period
of growing beyond a connection with the physical body or with physical
existence in general—of shedding the habit of it.

We know that after passing through the gateway of death our astral
body initially still possesses all the powers that were present in it at the
moment of death. We have only laid aside the physical body, the
instrument of enjoyment and action: we no longer possess it, but do still
have the astral body as the bearer of passions, drives, desires and
instincts. After death—out of habit you might say—we still long for
precisely the same things that we longed for during life. In life, of
course, we satisfy our longings and desires through the instrument of
the physical body. Without this instrument after death we lack all
possibility of satisfying such things. We experience this as a kind of
thirst for physical life until we have become accustomed to living only in
the spiritual world as such, and possessing only what derives from the
world of spirit. Until we have learned this, we sojourn in the period we
refer to as that of weaning from our habits, the period of kamaloca.

In describing the very distinctive course of this process we saw that
human life runs backwards during this time. This is extremely hard for
someone new to spiritual science to understand. We pass backwards
through the kamaloca period—which takes around a third of the length
of our previous life. Let us assume that someone dies at the age of 40. He
passes through all the events he experienced in life in reverse sequence.
Thus he first experiences what happened when he was 39, followed by
38, 37, 36 and so on. He passes through his life backwards to the
moment of his birth. On this is based the beautiful Christian saying
referring to the moment when human beings re-enter the world of spirit
or the kingdom of heaven, 'Except ye become as little children, ye shall
in no wise enter the kingdom of heaven.'[48] In other words, we live our
way back to the time of childhood, and re-experience it; and having

completed this reverse journey, we enter devachan or the kingdom of heaven, and there spend the rest our time in the spiritual world. This is hard to picture, since we are so used to the course of time on the physical plane being an absolute reality. It takes some effort therefore for us to find our way into such ideas. But this gradually becomes possible.

Now we must call to mind what we actually do in kamaloca. Naturally we could offer many varied descriptions, but today let us focus on something that relates directly to our question about the karmic cause of illnesses. What will be said here should certainly not be seen as the only mode of experiencing kamaloca, but as one among many.

First we can illustrate how this kamaloca period is used to serve our future by imagining that the person who died at the age of 40 did something at the age of 20 that harmed another. Whenever we do something that harms someone else, this has a certain significance for the whole of life. Anything we do that harms a fellow human being or another creature, or the world in general, represents a developmental hindrance, an obstacle to our developmental progress. This is the whole meaning in fact of our human pilgrimage: the founding power of the human soul, passing from one incarnation to another, is at all times geared to progressive development and strives for higher evolution. But as we evolve we repeatedly place obstacles in our own path, as it were. If this fundamental power—which is what seeks to respiritualize the soul—were active on its own, a very brief period on earth would be sufficient for us. But in that case the whole of earthly evolution would have taken a quite different course, and the purpose of it would not be achieved. It is only by placing obstacles in our own path that we gain strength and gather experience.

By placing obstacles in our own path, and then eradicating and overcoming these again, will we become the strong being that we must become by the end of earthly evolution. It is absolutely part of the meaning of Earth evolution for us to place obstacles in our own path. And if we did not have to acquire the strength to remove the hindrances again, we would not develop the strength we need. In other words, the world would be deprived altogether of the strength which we develop in this way. We have to overlook entirely the good and bad connected with such hindrances. From the very beginning, the wise guidance of the world sought to enable human beings to place obstacles in their own path so that they might remove them again and thus develop the great strength for what would come later in the world. One might even say that this wise guidance allowed the human being to be evil, gave him the opportunity to be so, to do harm, so that, by redressing the harm, overcoming the evil, he would grow into a stronger being during karmic evolution than he otherwise would have become if he had effortlessly attained his goal. This is how we must regard the meaning and justification of such obstacles and hindrances.

So when, after death, someone lives backwards through his life in kamaloca and arrives at any harm he has done, say an injury he did to someone when he was 20, he experiences this harm in the same way that he re-experiences the joy and goodness which he gave others. But in this case he experiences within his own astral body the pain he inflicted. So let us assume he struck someone when he was 20, and the other suffered the pain of this blow. As he lives back through his experiences, he feels in his astral body the very pain he caused, which the other experienced when he received the blow. In the world of spirit, therefore, we pass objectively through everything that we ourselves caused in the outer world. By this means we absorb the strength, the tendency to redress this pain in one of our subsequent incarnations. In retracing our experience after death we register in our own astral body what it felt like to be on the receiving end of what we did. And we also register how in doing this we placed a stone in the path of our own further development. The stone must be removed! Otherwise we cannot advance beyond it. At this moment we form the intention, the tendency, to remove the stone. And so when we have passed through the kamaloca period we actually arrive in the period of our childhood with pure intentions—that is, with the intention of removing all the hindrances we ourselves created in life. The fact that we bear these intentions within us leads to the unique configuration of each person's future biography.

Let us assume that, at the age of 20, B did A an injury. Now he must experience the pain of it himself, and he takes with him the intention to make amends to A in a future life—in the physical world, since that is where the injury occurred. The fact that he bears within him the strength—that is the will—to make amends creates a bond of attraction between B and A, to whom the injury was done. In the next life this bond of attraction leads them together again. The mysterious power of attraction that leads people together in life originates in what was absorbed in kamaloca and the powers developed there. During life we are led to the people to whom we need to make reparation, or with whom we have had anything at all to do by virtue of what we underwent in kamaloca. Now you can imagine that what we absorbed as the kamaloca powers of redress for one life cannot by any means always make amends in one single further life. It may be that we formed a large number of connections with people in one life, and that the subsequent kamaloca period gave us the opportunity to encounter these people again. But it also depends on these others whether we again form connections with them in our subsequent life. It can be spread over many lifetimes. In one life we need to make redress for this, in another for something else, and so on. We should not think that we can immediately make amends in our next life for everything in this one. This depends on whether the other person also develops a corresponding attraction for us in his soul.

Let us now examine the workings of karma in more detail, in relation to a particular instance. In kamaloca we form the intention of carrying out something in our next life, or one of our next lives. The powers implanted in our soul remain there, do not disappear again. We are reborn with all the powers that we have absorbed. This is completely unavoidable. Now in life we are not just faced with things that must be done to make karmic redress, although what I am about to say can also relate to that. We have placed various kinds of obstacle in our path, have lived in a one-sided way, have failed to make proper use of our life, have pursued only one or another sort of enjoyment, one or another kind of work. In other words we have let other opportunities that life offered pass us by, thus failing to develop other capacities. This too awakens karmic causation in us in kamaloca.

Thus we enter into our next life, are born aged nought. Now let us assume that we live to the age of 10, 20. In our soul lie all the kamaloca powers we absorbed, and these emerge when they have grown ripe for life. At a certain period of our life an inner need or urge will invariably arise to enact such an impulse. Let us assume that at 20 an inner urge arises in us to perform a particular deed because we absorbed this power in kamaloca. Let's stay with this, since it is the simplest example: an inner urge arises to make amends to someone. The person in question is there, the bond of attraction has led us to him. External factors certainly allow us to do this. But a hindrance can still exist: the redress might demand a deed of us that is beyond the capacities of our organism. Our constitution and organism is also dependent on the forces of heredity, and this always causes disharmony in every life. When we are born we are, on the one hand, embedded in the forces of heredity. The physical body and ether body inherit the qualities that the genetic line can bequeath us. This legacy is of course not entirely devoid of all outward connection with our soul's karmic intentions. You see, as our soul descends from the world of spirit it is drawn to the parents, to the family where qualities are passed down that are most closely related to the soul's needs. But they are never fully commensurate with these needs—the body cannot match this. There is always a certain discrepancy between inherited forces and what the soul bears within it from its past life. And ultimately it is a question of whether the soul is strong enough to overcome all resistance present in the genetic line, and can elaborate the organism throughout life in such a way as to overcome what is not suited to it. People vary a great deal in this respect. There are souls whose past lives have made them very strong. Such a soul must be born into the body best fitted for it, but not into a perfectly suitable body. The soul can be strong enough more or less to overcome everything that does not accord with it, but this may not always be the case. Let us examine this in detail, considering our brain in this respect.

We inherit this instrument of our life of ideas and thinking from our ancestors as an external instrument. Its finer curvatures and convolutions have been shaped in a particular way in the line of descent. To a certain degree the soul's inner power will always be able to overcome what does not suit it, and adapt its tool to its own forces—but only up to a certain point. A stronger soul can do this more, a weaker soul less. And if prevailing circumstances even mean it is impossible for our soul forces to overcome the brain's resistant disposition and organization, then we cannot properly use this instrument. Our incapacity to make full use of this instrument manifests as a mental deficiency, or so-called mental illness. When the powers of the soul are not strong enough to overcome certain traits of our organism, what we call a melancholic temperament can also develop. So now, at the midpoint of incarnation—things are different at the beginning and end of life—we always have in us a certain discrepancy between the instrument and the soul forces, and this is invariably the secret cause of inner ambivalence and disharmony in human nature. Everything a person will often consider to be the cause of his dissatisfaction is usually only a mask. In truth the causes lie elsewhere, as I have just suggested. And so we see how the soul, living on from incarnation to incarnation, interacts with what we receive through the line of heredity.

Now let us imagine that we have been reborn and that, at the age of 20, our soul feels the urge to make amends for some action or other. The person in question is also there, but our soul is incapable of overcoming the inner resistance in a way that could allow the deed to be performed. After all, we always have to set our powers in motion in order to perform any action. People usually do not notice that something is occurring within them, and do not initially need to notice. The following may certainly happen. A person lives in the world. In his soul, 20 years after his birth, lives the urge and drive to make amends in some way. The possibility of doing so exists, and external circumstances allow it. But inwardly he is incapable of using his organs in a way that would enable him to realize the action he should carry out.

A person need not know anything of what has been said here but he will become aware of its effect, which arises as some form of illness—and here we find the karmic connection between what happened in a former life and illness. Given this spiritual causation, the whole disease process will be such as to render the person capable of making amends, of strengthening him sufficiently to do so, whenever circumstances allow this again. Thus at the age of 20 we may be unable to perform this or that restorative action. But the drive or urge is there, and the soul desires to do it. What does the soul do instead? It battles with its unyielding organ, taking up arms against it, and the result is that it lays waste to it as it were, destroys it. The organ that ought really to be used to perform an outward deed is destroyed under the influence of these forces, and this leads in turn to a reaction process which we can now regard as the process of healing. The organism's powers must be invoked to rebuild the organ. This organ that has been laid waste, because it was not as it should have been to allow the person to undertake the work he needed to, is reconfigured through the illness in line with the soul's requirements in order to perform the deed in question. In some circumstances it will be too late after the illness for the deed to be accomplished. But the soul has now taken up a quite different power so that when it reincarnates it will configure the organ through growth and overall development to enable it to accomplish the deed. Thus illness can endow us in one life with the strength and capacity to realize our karmic obligations in a next.

Here we have a mysterious connection between illness, which is basically a process that furthers upward evolution, a karmic connection between illness and this ascending evolution. In order for the soul to develop the strength to allow an organ to be configured in the way necessary for its use, this unsuitable organ must be broken down and rebuilt by soul forces. Here we meet a law that applies to human bio-graphy and that must be roughly defined as follows: we need to acquire strength by gradually overcoming resistance we encounter in the phy-sical world. Basically we have gained all the powers we possess by overcoming one or another kind of resistance in former lives. The capacities we have today result from our illnesses in former lives.

To be quite clear about this, let us imagine that a soul is not yet capable enough of using the midbrain. By what means can it acquire the capacity to make proper use of the midbrain? Only by previously observing this incapacity, breaking down the organ and then recon-figuring it. As the soul reshapes it, it learns to acquire the specifically oriented power that it needs. We possess as capacity everything which we ourselves have in the past undertaken through destruction and re-synthesis. This has been sensed by all world faiths that assigned a very significant being to the process of destruction and re-creation. In Indian religion, 'Shiva' embodies the powers that preside over destruction and re-creation.

Here already we have one of the ways in which you can say that processes of illness are karmically induced. Something like this, whereby

diseases appear in a more general form, certainly obtains for the processes in which the more general nature of the human being is involved,
as opposed to the human individuality. For instance, we see the typical
childhood illnesses arise at certain times. These are nothing other than
an expression of the fact that the child learns to inwardly master certain
organs in childhood illnesses, and will then be able to govern them in all
following incarnations. We should regard illnesses as a process that
renders us stronger and more capable. Here we come to a quite different
way of thinking about illnesses. Naturally we should not apply the same
explanation to someone who is run over by a train. The explanation for
all such things must invariably be sought in a realm separate from
disease, separate from what I have just characterized. However, there is
another instance of karmic causation of illness that is no less interesting
and that we can also only understand if we characterize life circumstances in somewhat more detail.

Imagine that you learn some kind of lesson in life. First you have to
learn it, since the most important acquirements in life are certainly first
learned. The process of learning is an absolutely necessary one. But this
is never the whole story, since learning itself is only the most external
process. Having integrated something into ourselves, having learned
whatever the lesson is, we still have a long way to go before experiencing
all that these lessons must fulfil in us. We are born into life with very
specific capacities, partly acquired through heredity and partly through
our former lives. The scope of our capacities is limited. In each life we
increase the sum of our experiences. What we experience and undergo is
not connected with us in the same way as what we bring into our life as
innate temperament, natural predisposition and so forth. What we have
learned during life initially as memory and habit is more loosely connected with us. In life therefore it also appears in isolated aspects. Only
after life does it emerge in the ether body, the great memory tableau.
We must now incorporate it into us; it must be added to our being.

So let us assume that we have learned something in our life and are
then reborn. Due to heredity or other circumstances, also perhaps
because our learning did not develop harmoniously and though we
learned one thing or another we did not learn what we needed to bring
our learning to full fruition—it may very well be that when we are

reborn we will develop what we learned in a particular direction, but not in another. Let us assume we learned something in one life that in the next required a particular part of our brain to be organized in this or that fashion, or our blood circulation to run in a certain way, and then imagine also that we did not learn the other things necessary to complement this. This will not by any means necessarily lead directly to any apparent defect in us. We have to progress erratically in our lives, experiencing and coming to perceive that we have pursued something in a one-sided way. Now, when we are reborn with the fruits of what we learned, we lack the capacity to elaborate it all in ourselves in a way that allows it to be realized or enacted. For instance, someone may even have gained some degree of initiation into the great secrets of existence during one incarnation. When reborn, these powers implanted in him will seek to emerge. But let us assume he has been unable to develop certain powers that can then produce the appropriate harmony in his organs. At a certain point in his life what he previously learned will certainly seek to emerge. But he lacks an organ that would be necessary to realize this. What is the consequence of this? An illness must develop, one whose karmic cause may lie very, very deep. And again we can say that a part of the organism must be broken down and reconfigured. Then, in this reconfiguration, the soul senses the new direction for the right powers, and takes with it this sense of what the right powers are. If this originates in such learning or even initiation, however, it is usually the case that the fruits appear in this same life. Here an illness manifests in a way that enables the soul to sense that it lacks something specific. And then, for instance, immediately after the illness, something can arise that would not otherwise have been accessible to us. It may be that in the previous life we could have risen to a certain degree of spiritual enlightenment, but now a node or point in the brain has not opened— we have not developed the power allowing us to open it. It is then inevitable that this node must be destroyed, and this can lead to a grave illness. Then the relevant part is re-formed and as this happens the soul senses the powers necessary for it to open; and subsequently the destined enlightenment occurs. We can certainly regard processes of illness as significant heralds.

Here however we encounter things that our mundane world dismisses out of hand. Nevertheless, it is not an uncommon experience for someone to feel continual dissatisfaction—as though something exists in the soul that cannot emerge, and makes life more or less inwardly impossible. Then a grave illness arrives, the overcoming of which leads to entirely new conditions, acting like redemption: a node is opened and the organ can be used. The sense of dissatisfaction was due only to the fact that the organ could not be used. In fact, people have many such 'nodes' in their current cycle of life, and they cannot all be opened. This is not invariably a matter of gaining enlightenment but can manifest in many secondary life processes.

Thus we find ourselves confronting the need to develop this or that aspect, and can see that a cause of illnesses lies here too, in the karmic chain of causation. This is why we should never really be entirely satisfied with a merely trivial view of illness as something we attract to ourselves through karma. This is because we ought not merely to consider the karma of the past, thus seeing an illness as a conclusion, but instead regard illness—which is only a secondary phenomenon—as the developing cause of our future creative power and capacity. We misunderstand illness and karma entirely if we always only consider the past, thereby making karma a more or less completely random law of destiny. Karma becomes a law of action, of life's fruitfulness, however, if we are able to look through the lens of present karma into the future.

All this points to a great law that holds sway in our human existence. And in order to gain at least a faint intimation of this great law—we will return to it later and describe it in more detail—let us cast our gaze back to the time when we first arose in our present human form, in the Lemurian era. At that time we descended from divine-spiritual existence into the external existence we know today, first embodying ourselves and thus embarking on the path of outward incarnations, then passing onwards from one incarnation to the next through to the present time. Before we embarked on our incarnations, the opportunity we have today for implanting illnesses in ourselves did not yet exist. Not until we acquired the capacity to regulate our relationship with our surroundings did it become possible for us to go astray, inducing mistaken inner organ configurations and implanting in ourselves the predisposition for disease. Prior to this it was impossible for the human being to produce processes of disease in himself. When everything was still subject to the sway of divine powers and forces, before our lives were in our own hands, no potential for illness as yet existed. Then this potential for illness developed. Where will we best learn to discover the paths of healing therefore? We will learn this best if we are able to look back to times when divine, spiritual powers worked into the human being, bestowing upon him absolute health unsullied by any possibility of disease—in other words before we first began to incarnate. Those who had some insight into these things always harboured such feelings. From this starting point, try to engage deeply with mythological narratives and images. At present I am not even referring to the true source of healing lore in the Egyptian rites of Hermes, but only to the Greek and Roman Asclepius rites.

One can say that Asclepius, the son of Apollo, is the father of Greek physicians. And what does the Greek myth tell us about him? As a youth, Asclepius's father brought him to the mountains to be apprenticed to the centaur Chiron. This centaur, Chiron, instructs Asclepius, the father of medicine, in the healing powers of herbs and other medicinal forces to be found on the earth. What kind of creature is the centaur Chiron? He is described as one who existed before Lemurian times, before humanity's descent to earth, a being who is half man, half animal. This myth conceals the fact that Asclepius was initiated in the relevant mysteries into the great powers of health, the great health-bestowing powers, before human beings embarked on their first incarnation.

And so we find an expression in Greek myth of this great law, this great spiritual reality, which is of such interest to us in relation to humanity's earthly pilgrimage. Myths are in reality images of life's profoundest relationships, and will reveal their depths once we get a little further than the ABC of spiritual science. Myths, particularly, are images of the deepest secrets of human existence.

If all of life is considered from this perspective, then all of life, likewise, will be seen in its light, and spiritual science will increasingly become something—and we must increasingly emphasize this—that will find its way into ordinary daily life. People will come to *live* spiritual science, thus realizing what has in fact been the guiding aim of spiritual science from the very outset. Spiritual science will become the great impulse for humanity's ascent, for the true redemption and progress of humanity.

LECTURE 15

A lecture given here about more complex questions of reincarnation[49] will have allowed you to see that initial, elementary truths of spiritual science are modified as we gradually rise to insight into ever higher worlds. It is nevertheless right to represent general, universal truths in as elementary and simple a way as possible at the beginning; but at the same time we need gradually to leave our ABC primers behind us and work our way through to higher truths. You see, these higher truths are what gradually enable us to accomplish something that is part of spiritual science's intended gift to us: the capacity to understand and penetrate the world that surrounds us in the sensory, physical domain. There is of course a long way still to go in this ascending journey before we succeed in drawing the lines and forces underlying the world of the senses into an overall context of some kind. Yet many things that have been said in recent sessions will have helped one or another aspect of our existence to become clearer and more explicable. Today we will try to go a little further and again speak of more complex questions of reincarnation.

To do so we need to clarify, above all, that beings who hold a leading position in the evolution of humanity on earth differ from one another. In the course of our earthly evolution we must distinguish leading individualities who have, one can say, evolved with the humanity of our earth from the beginning, albeit advancing more quickly than us. We could put it like this: if we look back to our long-distant Lemurian past, we find the most varied degrees of evolution amongst the human beings incarnated at that time. All the souls incarnated, embodied at that time, passed through repeated incarnations throughout the subsequent Atlantean period and then our post-Atlantean era. Souls evolved at different speeds, and here we find those who evolved relatively slowly through different incarnations and will still need to pass through long, long evolutionary journeys in future. There are also, though, other souls who evolved rapidly and who, you can say, used their incarnations more productively and therefore today stand at a level of soul-spiritual, and thus spiritual development so advanced, that an ordinary modern person will only achieve it in the very far distant future. But staying in this sphere of souls, we can say that however advanced such souls may be, however lofty they may be compared to ordinary people, they underwent the same earthly evolution as others, and simply advanced more quickly.

Apart from these leading individualities, who are kindred with other human beings but just stand at a higher level, there are other individualities, other beings who, as humanity evolved, certainly did not pass through different incarnations as the others did. We can roughly illustrate what underlies this if we consider that in the Lemurian times we have been studying, beings existed who no longer needed to descend so deeply into physical embodiment as other human beings, as all the beings that have been described. These were therefore beings who could have pursued their evolution into higher, more spiritual regions, and whose own further progress did not necessitate them descending into bodies of flesh. But a being of this kind can nevertheless intervene in the course of human evolution by, as it were, vicariously descending into a body of the kind human beings have. Thus at some point or other a being, an entity, can appear; and if we study such a being's soul clairvoyantly, we can establish that it is not one who can be traced back in time as others can: that we cannot find a succession of previous physical incarnations. In tracing this soul back through time we may not find any former bodily incarnation whatsoever. If we do discover a physical embodiment, then it is basically only because such beings can also frequently descend and incarnate vicariously in a human body. A spiritual being of this kind, one therefore who descends into a human body in order to intervene in evolution as a human being, gains no advantage from this incarnation, finds no personal meaning in experiences acquired here in the world. In the eastern tradition, such a being is called an 'avatar'. And that is the difference between a leading being emerging from human evolution as such and one called an avatar: that the latter draws no fruits from the physical incarnations, or incarnation, which he undergoes, since he enters a physical body for the purpose of bringing salvation and progress to human beings. To sum up, such an avatar can enter a human body on one or more occasions, yet will be decidedly different from any other human individuality.

As you will gather from the spirit of all the lectures given here, the greatest avatar being who has lived on earth is Christ, the being we designate as Christ, who took possession of the body of Jesus of Nazareth when the latter was 30 years of age. This being, who first came into contact with our earth two millennia ago, was incarnated in a body of flesh for three years. Since then he has been bound up with the astral sphere, thus with the spiritual sphere of our supersensible world. This avatar being is of wholly unique significance. We would seek the Christ being in a former human incarnation on earth in vain, although other, lower avatars can incarnate frequently. The difference does not lie in the fact that they incarnate often but that they draw no benefit for themselves from their earthly embodiments. Human beings give nothing to the world but only take from it, while these beings only give and take nothing from the earth. But if you wish properly to understand these things you will need to distinguish between an avatar as lofty as Christ was and lower avatar beings.

Such avatar beings can have the most varied missions on our earth. We can outline the kinds of mission they have, and to avoid skirting round the theme in a speculative way let us immediately take a specific instance and illustrate the possible nature of such a task.

You all know from the group of tales surrounding Noah[50] that ancient Hebrew texts assign a large portion of post-Atlantean, post-Noah humanity to three progenitors, Shem, Ham and Japheth. Today we are not going to enter further into what Noah and these three progenitors can tell us in a different context. We will just clarify the fact that Hebrew texts which refer to Shem, one of Noah's sons, see Shem as progenitor of the whole semitic line. A truly esoteric view of such matters, of such a tale, will discover the deeper truths underlying it. Those capable of studying such matters esoterically know the following about Shem, this progenitor of the Semitic race. From birth onwards, indeed even earlier, measures must be taken to ensure that such an individual, destined to be the progenitor of a whole line of descent, can actually fulfil this mission. What are these measures ensuring that Shem—in this example—can become the progenitor of a whole people or race? In Shem's case this occurred by means of him receiving, you can say, a very specially prepared ether body. When we are born, as you know, our ether or life body is incorporated around our individuality, alongside the other aspects of our human nature. For the ancestor of a whole race, a special ether body must be prepared and will act as pattern and archetype for the ether bodies of all future descendants of this individual in further generations. Such a progenitor, therefore, will have a typical ether body, a kind of matrix ether body; and then, through blood kinship this is passed on through the generations so that, in a sense, the ether bodies of all descendants belonging to the same line are reflections of the ancestor's ether body. All the ether bodies of the Semitic race, therefore, were interwoven with something like an image of Shem's ether body. How does such a thing occur during the course of human evolution?

If we take a closer look at this figure of Shem, we find that his ether body retained its archetypal form by virtue of the fact that an avatar wove himself into it. While not as lofty in nature as some others, this was nevertheless a high avatar being who descended into Shem's ether body. The avatar did not connect with either the astral body or the I of Shem, only as it were interweaving with his ether body. In this example we can already study the significance of an avatar participating in the human form and constitution. What is the overall meaning and purpose of a person such as Shem, whose mission is to be the progenitor of the whole race, having an avatar interwoven with his body? The significance of this is that each time an avatar is woven into a human being of flesh and blood some aspect or several aspects of this human being can multiply and replicate, can be split into numerous parts.

By virtue of the fact that an avatar was interwoven with Shem's ether body, it was possible for numerous copies of the original to arise, so that these countless copies could be woven into all those who descended from the progenitor over many generations. Thus the significance of an avatar's descent is, among other things, that it allows replication of one or several aspects of the being ensouled by the avatar. Countless copies of the original arise, all formed in its image. As you can gather, an especially valuable ether body was present in Shem, an archetypal ether body prepared and then woven into Shem by a high avatar so that it could descend in many replicated copies to all those who were to be related by blood to this ancestor.

In the lecture I referred to at the start, we also spoke of the fact that a spiritual economy exists, of a kind that preserves something of particular value and carries it on into the future. We have heard that the astral body and ether body can reincarnate as well as the I. Apart from the fact that countless copies of Shem's ether body arose, his own ether body was preserved in the spiritual world since it was of very great use in the later mission of the Hebrew people. All the distinctive characteristics of the Hebrew people had originally come to expression in this ether body. If something of very special importance should occur for the ancient Hebrew people—say the entrusting of a special mission or task—this could best be undertaken by an individual who bore within him this ether body of the progenitor.

This is indeed what occurred: an individuality who was later to intervene in the history of the Hebrew people bore the progenitor's ether body in him. Indeed, we have here one of those wonderful complications in humanity's evolution that can be so illuminating. A very high individuality, he had as it were to stoop down to the Hebrew people so as to be able to speak to them in a way they could understand, and give them the power to undertake a special mission. This was somewhat like a person of outstanding intellectual capacities learning the language of an untutored tribe in order to be able to communicate with them. He will not necessarily gain much himself by learning this language, but must adapt his thoughts to express them by this means, must make himself at home in the language. In a similar way, a high individuality had to adapt to and make himself at home in Shem's ether body in order to be able to bring a very specific impulse to the ancient Hebrew people. This is the figure named Melchizedek in biblical history. He clothed himself in Shem's ether body, as it were, to give Abraham the impulse that you will find described in the Bible. Thus apart from what was contained in Shem's individuality multiplying by virtue of an avatar incarnated in him and then being woven into all the other ether bodies of members of the Hebrew people, Shem's own ether body was preserved in the spiritual world so that Melchizedek could later wear it and thus pass on an important impulse to the Hebrew people via Abraham.

So finely woven are the realities underlying the physical world, and only through these we can understand what occurs in the physical world. We can only gain insight into history by grasping realities of a spiritual nature underlying physical realities. If we remain with merely physical realities, history—simply on its own terms—can never be understood.

What has been outlined here—the descent of an avatar leading to replication of the supersensible bodies of the one who bears this avatar within him, and the passing on to others of these copies of the archetype—is of very particular importance when we come to Christ's appearance on earth. By virtue of the fact that the avatar being of Christ dwelt in the body of Jesus of Nazareth, it became possible for both Jesus' ether body and astral body to be multiplied countless times. Even the I, as well, could be reproduced—as an impulse kindled in the astral body when the Christ entered the threefold aspects of Jesus of Nazareth. Initially though, we will consider how the avatar multiplied Jesus of Nazareth's ether body and astral body.

One of the most incisive moments in humanity's history occurs when the Christ principle appears within Earth evolution. What I have told you about Shem is basically typical and characteristic of the pre-Christian era. When an ether body, or also an astral body, is replicated in this way, its copies usually pass to those who are related by blood to the progenitor possessing its archetype. Thus copies of Shem's ether body were passed on to members of the Hebrew people. This changed when the Christ avatar appeared. The ether body and astral body of Jesus of Nazareth were multiplied, and these replicated copies were preserved until such time as they could be used in the course of humanity's evolution. But they were not tied to one or another nationality, tribe or race. Instead, in subsequent times, whenever a person appeared who was mature enough, who irrespective of his nationality was suited to receive a copy of Jesus of Nazareth's astral or etheric body, then this could happen, and these copies were woven into his own astral or ether body. We see the potential therefore for all kinds of people to have woven into them copies, like imprints, of Jesus of Nazareth's astral or ether body.

The intimate history of Christian evolution is connected with this fact. What is normally presented as Christian history is a sum of only external processes. And much too little attention is given, therefore, to the most important aspect—the distinguishing of real periods in Christian development. Those able to gain deeper insight into the evolution of Christianity will easily discover that the way in which Christianity was disseminated in the first Christian centuries was quite different from later centuries. In the earlier Christian period, the spread of Christianity was bound up with everything that could be acquired from the physical plane. We need only survey the early Christian teachers to find accentuation of physical memories, physical circumstances and everything physical that had been preserved. You need only recall that Irenaeus,[51] who made a major contribution to the spread of Christianity in different countries in the first century AD, placed great emphasis on the fact that in living memory people had witnessed the Apostles' pupils at first hand. Great importance was placed on being able to authenticate physical memories such as that Christ himself had taught in Palestine. That Papias[52] had himself sat at the feet of the Apostles was a matter of great importance. Even the dwelling places of those who had been eyewitnesses of Christ in Palestine were identified and described. Thus memory of these physical narratives was especially stressed in the first Christian centuries.

The extent to which all remaining physical evidence is accentuated can be seen in the words of Augustine of Hippo,[53] who lived at the end of this period, and stated: 'Why do I believe in the truths of Christianity? Because the authority of the Catholic Church compels me to.' For him, the key thing is the physical authority of something existing in the physical world: the corporeal reality in the linking of one person to another that can be followed back to someone like Peter as a companion of Christ. This is the decisive thing for him. So we can see that great worth is assigned to documents, to impressions gained from the physical plane in the first centuries of the spread of Christianity.

After Augustine's time through to around the tenth, eleventh and twelfth centuries things change in this respect: it is no longer possible to rely on living memory and only to cite physical evidence, since this lies in a past that is now too long gone. In the whole mood and outlook, too, of those who profess Christianity—and this is particularly true of people in Europe—something quite different is present. At this time something like direct knowledge of Christ's existence prevails, a knowledge that Christ died on the Cross and lives on. Between the fourth and fifth centuries and the tenth to twelfth centuries a great number of people would have considered it very misguided indeed to cast any doubt on the events in Palestine, for they knew better. Such people lived throughout Europe especially. They were always able to have something like a small-scale inner Pauline revelation, an experience of what Paul, who had previously been Saul, underwent on the road to Damascus—which transformed him into Paul.

What was it that enabled a number of people to receive something resembling clairvoyant revelations about the events of Palestine? This was possible because in these centuries the preserved copies or imprints of the replicated ether body of Jesus of Nazareth were woven into a large number of people. You can say that they were permitted to clothe themselves with these copies. Their ether body was not composed entirely of this image of Jesus' ether body but woven into their ether body was an image of the original that stemmed from Jesus of Nazareth. During these centuries there were people with the capacity to possess such an ether body, enabling them to have direct knowledge of Jesus of Nazareth and also of Christ. But this also meant that the image of Christ was released from external historical, physically conveyed tradition. It appears in a form most liberated from this tradition in the wonderful poem of the ninth century known as the Heliand Poem,[54] originating in the time of Louis the Pious, who ruled from 814 to 840. An outwardly plain and simple man in Saxony recorded it in writing. His astral body and I were far from equal to what his ether body contained, for this was interwoven with an image of Jesus of Nazareth's ether body. This humble Saxon pastor who wrote the poem down knew from direct clairvoyant perception, with great certainty, that Christ is present on the astral plane, and is the same who was crucified at Golgotha! And because he had direct and certain knowledge of this, he no longer needed to refer to historical documents. He no longer needed physical evidence that Christ had been there. He therefore describes him in a form emancipated from the whole setting of Palestine, released from the distinctive nature of Judaism. He describes him roughly as the lord of a Central European or Germanic tribe, and his adherents, the Apostles around him, as the thanes of a Germanic prince. All external scenes have been changed, retaining only the core, the eternal nature of the figure of Christ and the structure of events. Having this kind of direct knowledge, founded on something as immanent as an imprint of Jesus of Nazareth's ether body, this author did not have to lean upon actual historical events in speaking of Christ. Instead he dressed his direct knowledge in the garb of different outward surroundings. We find in this author of the Heliand Poem one of the remarkable individuals we described as possessing an ether body into which an imprint of Jesus of Nazareth's ether body was woven, and likewise we could find other such individuals at this period. Thus we see how something of the very greatest importance occurs behind physical events, and can offer us an intimate understanding of history.

Tracing Christian development further, we then come to the eleventh and twelfth centuries, through to the fifteenth. Here a quite different secret came into its own and carried the whole development further. Initially there was the memory of what occurred on the physical plane, then the etheric element wove itself directly into the ether bodies of Christianity's leading lights in Central Europe. In subsequent centuries, from the twelfth to the fifteenth century, the astral body of Jesus of Nazareth came to be woven in numerous images into the astral bodies of key sustainers of Christianity. Such people had an I that was capable of conceiving very mistaken ideas about all sorts of things; yet in their astral bodies lived an immediacy of power and devotion, and direct certainty of sacred truths. Such people possessed deep fervour, utter conviction and, in some circumstances, the capacity to substantiate this conviction. What can strike us sometimes as so strange in these individuals is the fact that their I was not equal to what their astral body contained—since the latter was interwoven with an imprint of the astral body of Jesus of Nazareth. The actions of their I sometimes seemed grotesque, contrasted with the majesty and lofty nature of the world of their feelings and moods, their religious fervour. Francis of Assisi[55] was one such individual. While we must have the deepest possible veneration for his whole world of feeling, for everything he did, the perspective outlined here can help us to understand things about his conscious I that seem incomprehensible to us today. He was one of those into whom was woven an imprint of the astral body of Jesus of Nazareth. And thus he was capable of accomplishing what he did. Numerous adherents of his in the Franciscan order, with its Servant Franciscans and Minorites, likewise had similar imprints woven into their astral bodies.

If you dwell properly, inwardly, on this world-evolutionary transition between past and future, then all the remarkable and otherwise strange and mysterious phenomena of those times can dawn clearly and brightly before you. We have to discern whether, woven into the astral bodies of these people of the Middle Ages, was more of what we call the sentient soul, or of the mind soul, or of the consciousness soul. The human astral body, you see, must in a sense be regarded as enclosing the I within it. Francis of Assisi was entirely imbued with what we can call the sentient soul of Jesus of Nazareth. And we can likewise experience the biographical trajectory of another wonderful personality in the most soulful way if we know the secret contained in her life: Elisabeth of Thuringia,[56] born 1207, was someone whose sentient soul was inwoven with an image of the astral body of Jesus of Nazareth. Knowing such a thing can resolve the riddle presented by such a figure.

And one particular phenomenon will become clear to you, above all, if you know that during this period the sentient soul, mind soul or consciousness soul, as imprints of the astral body of Jesus of Nazareth, were woven into many diverse individuals. The phenomenon I refer to is the discipline commonly called Scholasticism, something little understood today but much maligned. What task did Scholasticism set itself? It sought to draw on capacities of judgement and discernment, on the intellect, to find proofs and evidence for things for which neither a physical, historical basis existed nor which could any longer be perceived as direct, clairvoyant certainties—as had been possible in previous incarnations through the inwoven ether body of Jesus of Nazareth. The Scholastics set themselves a task based on the following insights: that tradition told them of the historical appearance of Christ Jesus, of the intervention in humanity's evolution of other spiritual beings of whom religious texts testify. Drawing on their rational or mind soul, on the intellectual aspect of the imprint of Jesus of Nazareth's astral body, they set themselves the task of proving, through subtle concepts that were clearly delineated and elaborated, all the mystery truths contained in their texts. Thus arose this remarkable discipline, an attempt to achieve acuity and intellectual prowess in a way probably unsurpassed in humanity's history. Over the course of several centuries—however you regard the *contents* of Scholastic thinking—the faculty of human reflection was nurtured and came to inform the whole culture of the age simply by virtue of the fact that concepts were defined, shaped and distinguished in such an extraordinarily subtle way. In the period between the thirteenth and fifteenth centuries, Scholasticism imprinted into humanity the faculty of thinking in acute and penetratingly logical ways.

In those informed more by the consciousness soul, or rather the manifesting imprint of the consciousness soul of Jesus of Nazareth, there appeared—since the I has its seat in the consciousness soul—the special insight that Christ can be found in the I. And since they themselves possessed the element of the consciousness soul from the astral body of Jesus of Nazareth, the inner Christ dawned in their inner life. Through this astral body they perceived that the Christ within them was the Christ himself. Meister Eckhart, Johannes Tauler[57] and all the key figures of medieval mysticism were of this kind.

You can see therefore how all successive phases of the astral body were replicated through the high avatar Christ entering the body of Jesus of Nazareth, and how they worked on in the subsequent period to bring about the actual development of Christianity. But there is yet another important transition. We see that humanity's development is also otherwise reliant on receiving and incorporating these aspects of the being of Jesus of Nazareth. In the first Christian centuries lived people wholly reliant on the physical plane; then came people in subsequent centuries who were predisposed to receive, woven into them, the element of Jesus of Nazareth's ether body. Later we can say that people were more oriented to the astral body, and it now also became possible for the imprint of Jesus of Nazareth's astral body to be incorporated into them. The astral body is the bearer of the power of judgement, which awoke most especially between the twelfth and the fourteenth centuries. You can gather this from yet another phenomenon as well.

Until this time it was quite clear to people how deep were the mysteries surrounding the Last Supper. All that lay in the words 'This is my body and this is my blood ...'[58] was accepted—at the most only debated in very small circles—as felt experience, because in these words Christ pointed to the fact that he will be united with the earth, with its planetary spirit. And since flour is the most precious substance derived from the physical earth, it became the body of Christ for people; and the sap that rises through plants, through the vine, came to contain something of the blood of Christ for them. This knowledge did not diminish the value of the Last Supper but, on the contrary, increased it. During these centuries people felt something of these endless depths, until the power of judgement awoke in the astral body. It is then that doubt also first arises; and from then on disputation about the Last Supper developed. Just consider the debates that went on among the Hussites, in the Lutheran faith and its factions under Zwingli and Calvin, about what the real nature of the Last Supper might be! Such debates would not have been possible formerly since people still retained direct knowledge of the Last Supper. But here we see demonstration of a great law of history, which is of particular importance for spiritual science: as long as people knew what the Last Supper was, they did not debate it. Only when they lost this direct understanding of the Last Supper did they enter into prolonged debate about it. You can take this as generally indicative of the fact that we do not really know the truth about something if we start discussing and debating it. Where knowledge exists, it is communicated, and really there will be little desire to debate it. Where desire for debate arises, there is usually no knowledge of the truth. Debate and dissent starts from lack of knowledge, and is invariably a sign of decline in understanding the serious core of a matter. A movement or cultural stream heads towards dissolution whenever debates commence. It is very important to repeatedly grasp the fact, in the domain of spiritual science, that the desire for debate can be regarded as a sign of lack of knowledge. By contrast we should cultivate the opposite of debate—which is the will to learn, the will gradually to gain insight into what is involved.

Here we see a great historical fact, verified in the development of Christianity itself. But we can learn something else if we see how the faculty of judgement, this acute, intellectual wisdom rooted in the astral body, develops during these centuries of Christianity. We must consider realities, not dogmas, however if we are to learn of all that Christianity progressively achieved. If we disregard the content of Scholasticism but focus on it as education and cultivation of capacities, we can ask what it later became. Do you know what it led to? Modern science! Modern science is inconceivable without the reality of this field of Christian scholarship in the medieval period. It is not just that Copernicus was a canon and Giordano Bruno a Dominican,[59] but that all the forms of thought which people used when getting to grips with the natural world from the fifteenth and sixteenth centuries onwards are nothing other than what was cultivated and nurtured between the eleventh and sixteenth centuries in medieval Christian scholarship. It is at odds with reality, is living in abstractions, to open Scholastic texts, compare them with those of modern science, and conclude that Haeckel et al. see things quite differently. We are concerned with realities here! Haeckel, Darwin, Du Bois-Reymond, Huxley[60] and others could never have written what they did without the precedents of medieval Christian scholarship. They owe the fact that they can think as they do to this scholarship, to Scholasticism. That is the reality. Through this schooling humanity learned to think in the true sense of the word.

We can pursue this further still. Read David Friedrich Strauss, and try to reflect on his mode of thinking. Try to be clear about his forms and configurations of thought—how he seeks to present the whole life of Jesus of Nazareth as a myth. Do you know where he gets his acuity of thinking? From medieval Christian scholarship. Everything used today to join such fierce battle with Christianity has been learned from medieval Christian scholarship. In fact it is true to say that no opponent of Christianity today could think as he does—and that therefore no such opponents could exist—if he had not learned such forms of thought from medieval Christian scholarship. A realistic appraisal of world history is however required to acknowledge this.

And what has actually happened since the sixteenth century? The I itself has increasingly come to the fore, and with it human egotism and, in turn, materialism. People have unlearned and forgotten all the content the I absorbed, and have therefore inevitably restricted themselves to what the I can observe, what the sensory apparatus can give to ordinary rationality. Only this has it been able to take with it into the human being's inner dwelling. A culture of egotism distinguishes post-sixteenth-century civilization. But what needs to enter this I now? Christianity underwent development in the external physical body, in the ether body, in the astral body, and worked its way up as far as the I. Within this I it must now absorb the mysteries and secrets of Christianity itself. After this I has learned to think for a while through Christianity and has applied its thoughts to the external world, it must now become possible to make the I into an organ receptive to Christ. The I must again discover the wisdom that is the primal wisdom of the great avatar, of Christ himself. And how must this come about? Through a spiritual-scientific deepening of Christianity. Carefully prepared through the three stages of physical, etheric and astral development, it is now important for the organ to open within the human being that enables him to look into his spiritual environment—the eye that Christ can open for him. Christ descended to the earth as the greatest avatar being. Let us attune to a perspective that seeks to regard the world as it can be regarded once we have taken Christ into ourselves. Then we will find our whole world-evolutionary path to be incandescent with the Christ being, pervaded by him. In other words, we can describe how the human physical body first developed gradually on old Saturn, and was joined by the ether body on old Sun, by the astral body on old Moon, and how the I entered us on earth. And then we will find that all this seeks the goal of our ever-increasing autonomy and individualization so that we can incorporate into earthly evolution the wisdom that streams from the sun to the earth. Christ and Christianity must in a sense become the focal point of the emancipated I of modern times, the centre of its perspective on the world.

And so you can see how Christianity gradually prepared the way for what it was to become. In its first centuries, Christians absorbed it with their physical cognitive capacities, then later with their etheric faculties and, through the medieval period, with their astral faculties of cognition. After this, the true form of Christianity was suppressed for a while until the three bodies had schooled the I during post-Christian development. But having learned to think and direct its gaze outward into the objective world, this I is now also ready to perceive in this objective world, in all phenomena, the spiritual realities so intimately bound up with the central being, the being of Christ, and to see Christ everywhere as the underlying foundation in the most diverse, manifold forms.

We thus arrive at the starting point of spiritual-scientific understanding of and insight into Christianity, and can discern the task, the mission assigned to this movement for spiritual insight. At the same time we can recognize the reality of this mission. Just as each person has a physical, etheric and astral body and I, and gradually ascends to ever greater heights, the same holds true of Christianity's historical development. We can say that Christianity likewise has a physical body, ether body, astral body and I—one capable even, as in our own times, of denying its own origin and wellspring. We can see how egotistic the I can become, generally, while at the same time retaining the capacity to also take up the true being of Christ within it and ascend to ever higher levels of existence. The human being as a single individual corresponds to the wider world both in terms of the latter's integral wholeness and the course of its historical development.

By looking at things in this way, from a spiritual-scientific perspective, a broad panorama of the future opens before us—and we find that this can engage our hearts and fill them with enthusiasm. Increasingly we come to understand what we must do, knowing also that we are not just feeling our way blindly. Our approach, you see, has not been to concoct ideas and try arbitrarily to project them upon the future, but instead to reach for and pursue the ideas which have slowly and gradually been prepared through centuries of Christian evolution. Just as the I must first appear and can only gradually evolve towards Spirit Self, Life Spirit and Spirit Man upon the preceding foundation of physical body, ether body and astral body, so modern human beings with their I configuration, with their modern thinking, have only been able to evolve from the astral, etheric and physical forms of Christianity. Christianity has become *I*. Just as real as this course of preceding evolution is the fact that humanity's I form, its I configuration, can only become apparent once the astral and etheric configurations of Christianity have evolved. In future Christianity will evolve further, and will come to offer us quite different things, so that Christian evolution and Christian ways of life will arise in a new form. The transformed astral body will manifest as the Christian Spirit Self, and the transformed ether body as the Christian Life Spirit. And in a luminous future perspective of Christianity the star of Spirit Man, towards which our lives slowly work their way, rises and shines before our souls as a radiant light, as the luminous spirit of Christianity.

LECTURE 16

TODAY we will consider the question of what modern people can actually gain from spiritual science as we understand it here. We will try to answer this by recalling various things we have become acquainted with during the past winter. Initially it might seem to us as if this spiritual science were a world-view similar to others current today. It would be easy to suppose that people try to solve the riddles of life by the most varied means at their disposal, through religion or science, to satisfy what is regarded as their thirst for knowledge, their intellectual curiosity, and that spiritual science is just another of the many modern world-views—whether they be called materialism, monism, spiritualism, idealism, realism and so forth. In this view, spiritual science is likewise just something that might satisfy intellectual curiosity. But this is not the case. Rather, we can say that what we acquire through spiritual science endows us with a positive, ongoing benefit for our lives, not merely satisfying our intellect, our thirst for knowledge, but coming to be a real factor in life. If we wish to understand this we will need to broaden our scope somewhat today. We will have to consider humanity's evolution from a very particular perspective. We have often done this before, but now let us look at this again from another point of view.

We have often looked back to times that preceded the great flood of Atlantis, when our forefathers—in other words our own souls—lived in our ancestors' bodies on the ancient continent of Atlantis between Europe, Africa and America. And we looked back to those still more ancient times which we call the Lemurian epoch, when the human souls now incarnated stood at a much lower level of existence than they do today. Let us look back to this period again now, seeing that we achieved our current level of sentient life, will life and intelligence, and indeed our whole form, by virtue of the fact that spiritual beings at a higher level than us in the universe helped form our earthly existence. We have often spoken of the particular spiritual beings who participated in this—of those we call Thrones, the Spirits of Wisdom, Spirits of Movement, of Form, of Personality and so on.

These are the great builders and architects of existence, beings who enabled our human race to advance gradually to the stage it has reached today. But now we must be very clear that spirits and beings other than those who advance human evolution also intervened. Beings that are hostile to the progressive spiritual powers intervened in certain ways. And for each of these epochs, both the Lemurian and the Atlantean, and also the post-Atlantean epoch in which we now live, we can identify the spiritual beings who presented hindrances—adversary spiritual beings hostile to those who wish only to help humanity advance.

In the Lemurian age, the first we will be concerned with today in relation to earth evolution, luciferic beings intervened in our development. They are in a sense hostile to the powers that in those times sought only to help humanity progress. In the Atlantean age, spirits of the figure we call Ahriman, or also Mephistopheles, opposed the progressive powers. To name them precisely, ahrimanic spirits, mephistophelian spirits are the ones called the spirits of Satan in medieval views, and these should not be confused with Lucifer.

In our own times, other spiritual entities will gradually exert an obstructive effect on progressive spirits—and we will return to speak of these later. First, though, let us ask what these luciferic spirits really brought about in the ancient Lemurian age.

Today we will consider all this from a quite specific point of view. Where, really, did the luciferic spirits intervene in ancient Lemurian times? You will best understand what is involved here if you cast your mind back once again to the way in which human beings evolved.

You know that the human being evolved on old Saturn when the Thrones poured out their own substance, laying down the first germ of the human physical body. We know that subsequently the Spirits of Wisdom on old Sun and the Spirits of Movement on old Moon implanted in him, respectively, the ether or life body and then the astral body. It was now the task of the Spirits of Form to endow the human being with the I on earth so that he could in a sense become independent by distinguishing himself from his surroundings. But despite becoming independent in relation to the external world surrounding them on earth, human beings would never have gained independence in relation to these Spirits of Form. They would have remained reliant on them, governed and guided by them as though pulled by strings. That this did not happen resulted from the, in some respects benevolent, effect of the luciferic beings' opposition to the Spirits of Form during Lemurian times. These luciferic beings gave us the prospect of our freedom, though at the same time also investing us with the capacity for evil, the possibility of deterioration into sensual passions and desires. Where, then, did these luciferic spirits intervene? They intervened in what was present, what we had most recently been endowed with—in the astral body that in those days was our inmost being in a certain respect. They gained a foothold in it, took possession of it. If these luciferic beings had not approached us, the Spirits of Form would otherwise have been the only ones to take possession of the astral body. They would have imprinted it with the powers that endow us with our human countenance, making us the image of God, the image of the Spirits of Form. The human being would have become all this but would have remained dependent during his lifetime on these Spirits of Form, and would have stayed so through all eternity.

Thus the luciferic beings insinuated themselves into the astral body, so that two types of being were now at work there: those who help the human being to progress and those who inhibit him in this unwavering advance but substitute for this an inwardly consolidated self-reliance. If the luciferic beings had not approached us, our astral body would have retained its state of innocence and purity. No passions would have arisen in us to make us desire things only found upon the earth. We can say that the luciferic beings made passions, drives and desires denser and lower in nature. In the absence of luciferic beings, humankind would have longed continually to ascend again to its home in spiritual realms from which it first descended. The human being would have felt no inclination towards what surrounds him on earth, could not possibly have become interested in earthly impressions. It was the luciferic spirits who awoke this interest in him. They drove him into the earthly sphere by occupying his inmost being, his astral body. But what prevented human beings from lapsing entirely from the Spirits of Form at that time or from higher spiritual realms in general? What was it that prevented them from falling entirely under the sway of their interest in and desire for the sensory world?

The spirits who enable us to progress reached for a remedy, which involved imbuing the human being with something that would not otherwise exist in him: they imbued him with sickness, suffering and pain. This became the necessary counterweight to the deeds of the luciferic spirits.

The luciferic spirits gave us sensual desire; the higher beings, by adding sickness and suffering to the array of sensual desires and sensory interests, introduced a remedy to prevent us falling entirely under the sway of this sensory world. Thus the world contains for us as much suffering and pain as mere interest in the physical, sensory world. These balance each other fully, with neither having the upper hand: the sum of sensual desires and passions is precisely matched by sickness and pain. This resulted from the mutual influence of the luciferic spirits and the Spirits of Form in Lemurian times. If these luciferic spirits had not come, we would not have descended as early as we did into the earthly sphere. Our passions and desires for the world of the senses also meant that our eyes were opened sooner to perceive the whole compass of sensory existence. If things had unfolded smoothly as the progressive spirits intended we would only have perceived our earthly surroundings from the middle of Atlantean times onwards. And we would have perceived them spiritually, not as we do today but such that our surroundings would everywhere have revealed themselves as the expression of spiritual beings. Because we were transposed prematurely into the earthly sphere, and our earthly interests and desires drew us downwards, things unfolded in a different way from what would otherwise have occurred in the middle of the Atlantean period.

Because of this, the ahrimanic spirits, whom we can also call mephistophelian spirits, interfered in the human faculty of seeing and understanding. In consequence we fell into error, into what can really first be called 'conscious sin'. The host of ahrimanic spirits acted upon us from the middle of Atlantean times. What was the nature of the seduction exerted on us by this host of ahrimanic spirits? They darkened our gaze so that we failed to look through the veil of what we regard as material substance in our surroundings to the spirit as the true foundations of materiality. If human beings saw the spirit in every stone, plant and animal, they could never have fallen into error and thus into evil. If the progressive spirits alone had worked upon us, we would have been preserved from the illusions to which we always succumb when we base everything on what the world of the senses tells us.

What remedy to this temptation was found by the spiritual beings who wish to support us in our progress and further development? How did they counter such error and sensory illusion? They took steps to enable us, now properly for the first time, to gain from the sensory world the possibility of overcoming error, sin and evil by bearing and working out our karma. Naturally this only occurred gradually, but the powers underlying this development originated here. Thus while beings called on to redress the seduction of luciferic beings introduced pain and suffering into the world—and of course also death which is related to it—those whose task it was to make good what results from error about the sensory world gave us the potential through our karma of dispelling all error again, of once more erasing all evil that we ourselves perpetrate in the world. What would have happened if we had irredeemably succumbed to evil and error? We would then have gradually united with this error, you can say, and have lost all capacity to develop further. You see, with every error, every lie, every illusion we throw an obstacle upon our further path. Our progress would always be pushed backwards by the obstacles of every error and sin if we were not capable of correcting these. In other words we would then actually be unable to reach the goal of human evolution. It would be simply impossible to attain humanity's goal if the restorative counter-forces of karma did not act.

Imagine for a moment that you do something wrong in one life. This wrong that you do, if it just stays there unremedied in your life, is tantamount to losing the forward step you would have taken if you had not committed the wrong. With every wrong or unjust act you do, you would lose a step forward, and these acts would all add up to retrogression, to slipping backwards. If there were no possibility of raising ourselves above error, we would ultimately get bogged down by it. But the boon of karma arose. How does this benefit us? Is karma something we should fear, should be frightened by? No, it is a power for which we ought actually to feel grateful to universal dispensation. You see, karma tells us that if we have done something misguided, mistaken, we must reap what we sow, for 'God is not mocked'.[61] The result of our error is that we must remedy it. Having done so we have excised it from our karma and can take further forward steps.

Without karma we could not possibly advance during our lives. Karma grants us the boon of requiring us to make good everything retrograde that we have done, to eradicate it again. Thus karma arose as the consequence of Ahriman's deeds.

And now let us delve further. In our time we are approaching an age when other beings will engage with us—beings who will increasingly intervene in the human future, the human evolution that still awaits us. Just as the luciferic spirits intervened in the Lemurian age, and the ahrimanic spirits in the Atlantean age, so beings will gradually also intervene in our own times. Let us be quite clear for a moment what kinds of being these will be.

The entities intervening in Lemurian times, as we saw, settled in the human being's astral body, drawing his drives and desires down into the earthly sphere. But to be more precise, what exactly did these luciferic beings settle in and fasten upon?

You will only be able to understand this if you recall the configuration of human nature as set out in my book *Theosophy*. There we find a necessary distinction, initially, between our physical body, ether or life body and our astral body or, as I have called it there, the sentient or soul body.

In studying these three aspects we find they are precisely the same as the three given us before we embarked on our lives on earth. What is referred to as the physical body acquired its initial form on old Saturn, while the ether body first developed on old Sun, and the soul or sentient body on old Moon. During our current Earth stage of evolution the sentient soul was gradually added as, really, an unconscious transformation or adaptation of the sentient body. Lucifer rooted himself in this sentient soul, insinuating himself into it and settling down there. There he sits. Then the mind soul developed also, through unconscious adaptation of the ether body. I have gone into greater detail on this in my treatise on *The Education of the Child*.[62] In this second aspect of the human soul, the mind soul—thus in the reworked part of the ether body—Ahriman rooted himself. There he sits, and leads humankind to false judgements about the material world, leads us into error, sins and lies, to everything in fact that derives from the rational or mind soul. For instance, whenever people embrace the illusion that matter is the be-all and end-all, this can be attributed to the suggestive influences of Ahriman, of Mephistopheles. The third in this progressive sequence is the consciousness soul, which consists of an unconscious reworking of the physical body. You will remember how this adaptation arose. Towards the end of Atlantean times, the head's ether body merged completely with the physical head, gradually transforming the physical body to make the human being a self-aware entity. Basically we are still working today on this unconscious adaptation of the physical body, on the consciousness soul. And in the forthcoming period, the spiritual beings called the Asuras will insinuate themselves into this consciousness soul and thus also into what we call the human I—for the I comes to expression in the consciousness soul. The Asuras will develop evil with an intensity far greater than did the satanic powers of the Atlantean age, or the luciferic spirits of Lemurian times.

The evil which the luciferic spirits brought upon us, at the same time as granting us the boon of freedom, is something we will shed entirely in the course of earthly evolution. The evil brought by the ahrimanic spirits can be dispelled in the unfolding of karmic lawfulness. But the evil which the asuric powers bring cannot be expunged in the same way. Whereas the good spirits brought us pain and suffering, illness and death so that we might evolve upwards despite our capacity for evil, and whereas they brought us the possibility of karmic redress to counterbalance ahrimanic powers and compensate for error, things will not be so straightforward in relation to the asuric spirits as earthly evolution progresses. This is because these asuric spirits take hold of our deepest, inmost being—the consciousness soul with the I—and cause this I to unite with the sensory, carnal nature of the earth. One portion of the I after another will be torn from it and, as the asuric spirits increasingly settle and take root in the consciousness soul, we will increasingly be obliged to leave parts of our existence behind on the earth. What succumbs to the asuric powers will be irretrievably lost. This does not mean that our whole being must succumb to them, but the asuric spirits will excise portions of the human spirit. In our age these Asuras are announcing themselves in the prevailing outlook we can call that of merely sensual life, the forgetfulness of all true spiritual beings, realities and worlds. We can say that so far the asuric temptation remains more theoretical. So far their deception is a widespread suggestion that the I is merely an outcome of the physical world alone, and their seduction one which leads people to a kind of theoretical materialism. But as things continue—and this is becoming increasingly apparent in the wasteland of sensory passions that rain down more and more upon earth—they will darken the gaze of humankind for spiritual beings and spiritual powers. People will know nothing and will not wish to know anything about a world of spirit. More than just *subscribing* to the doctrine that the loftiest ethical ideas are just highly developed animal drives, that human thinking is merely a transformation of animal senses, that in form we are closely related to animals and that our whole nature derives directly from them, human beings will come to *live* according to this view, will see themselves in this way and act accordingly.

Today, after all, no one actually lives as if their nature derives from animals. But this world-view will certainly come, and will result in people also really starting to live like animals, descending into merely animal instincts, drives and passions. And in some of the phenomena we need not describe further here, manifesting particularly as empty orgies of pointless sensuality that occur in large cities, we can see already the grotesque hell-fire of the spirits we call the Asuras.

Let us direct our gaze back in time once more. We saw that suffering, pain and also death were bestowed on us by the spirits who wish us to advance. In the Bible this is clearly announced in the phrase 'In pain thou shalt bring forth children ...'[63] Here death enters the world, and these things were a destiny brought upon us by the powers opposed to the luciferic. Who bestowed karma upon us, and who made it possible at all for karma to exist for us? You will only understand what is now said if you do not adhere pedantically to fixed concepts of earthly time. In terms of earthly time, people believe that whatever happens at any point can only cause an effect at a subsequent moment. But in the world of spirit, the effects of what happens are apparent beforehand; these effects already exist before their cause. To what is the boon of karma due? What did this benevolent deed of karma spring from in our earth's evolution? It comes from no other power in all evolution than from Christ.

Although Christ did not appear until a later time, he was always present in the earth's spiritual sphere. Already in the ancient Atlantean oracles, the priests of the oracle spoke of the spirit of the sun, of Christ. The Holy Rishis in the ancient Indian epoch spoke of Vishvakarman, and in Persia Zarathustra spoke of Ahura Mazda. Hermes spoke of Osiris; and Moses, the precursor and prophet of Christ, spoke of the power whose eternal nature counterbalances all the natural world—the power that lives in the *ehjey asher ehjey* (I am that I am).[64] All of them were speaking of Christ, but where was he to be found in these ancient times? Only where the eye of spirit could penetrate—the world of spirit. He was always present and active in, and from, the world of spirit. He it was who, before he ever appeared on earth, bestowed from above upon the human being the possibility of karma. Then he himself appeared on earth, and we know what he became for us through doing so. We have described his workings in the earthly sphere itself, and the significance of the event of Golgotha. We have also described his effects upon those who were not incarnated in an earthly body at the time the event of Golgotha occurred, but were then in the world of spirit. We know that at the moment when Christ's blood flowed from his wounds on Golgotha the spirit of Christ appeared in the underworld; and we saw that the whole world of spirit was lit up and illumined. We saw that Christ's appearance on earth is the most important event for the world, too, which we pass through between death and a new birth.

The effect that emanates from Christ is a thoroughly real one. We need only ask ourselves what would have happened to the earth if Christ had not appeared. The image of a Christ-less earth is one that can vividly show us the whole significance of Christ's appearance. Let us assume for a moment that Christ never appeared and the event of Golgotha did not occur. Before Christ's appearance, the souls of the most advanced human beings had acquired the profoundest interest in earthly life, and experienced the spiritual world in a way entirely in accord with the Greek saying 'Better a beggar in the upper world than a king in the world of shades'.[65] In the world of spirit, before the event of Golgotha, souls felt themselves alone and shrouded in obscurity. At that time the spiritual world was not transparent in its full, radiant clarity for those who passed through the gate of death and found themselves there. Each soul felt alone, isolated, as though surrounded by a wall that cut each off from the other. And this experience would have grown continually stronger. Human beings would have become hardened in their I, would have been completely thrown back on themselves, none finding the bridge to others. At each new incarnation, the egotism that already existed in great measure would have grown still more pervasive.

The whole of earth existence would have turned people increasingly into the crassest egotists. Nowhere on the globe would there have been any prospect whatever of a sense of fraternity or inner accord arising in human souls, for every passage through the spiritual realm would have reinforced and consolidated the ego. This is what would have happened on a Christ-less earth. We owe to Christ's appearance and the event of Golgotha the capacity of one soul to slowly find its way to the other, our capacity to include all humanity in the great encompassing power of fraternity. Thus Christ appears as the power who enables us to make proper use of earthly existence, or in other words to shape karma in a fitting way. Karma, you see, must be worked out on earth. To the workings of the Christ event, the presence of Christ in the earthly sphere, we owe our ability to find the strength to improve our karma as we should in earthly, physical existence and engage in ongoing further evolution.

Thus we see how the most diverse powers and beings work together in the course of humanity's evolution. Previously we only indicated in general that if Christ had not come to the earth humankind would have sunk into error. We can see in very clear, precise terms now that human beings would have grown inwardly ever harder, becoming something like self-enclosed spheres, globes, each for himself, and knowing nothing about other beings. Error and sin would have driven human-kind into this state.

Christ is the guiding light who leads us out of error and sin, and enables us to find the path of ascent. Now let us ask what human beings lost when they descended from the spiritual world and became enmeshed, under Lucifer's influence and then under Ahriman's influence, in error, illusion and lies in relation to the earthly world. They lost direct vision of the spiritual world, insight into and understanding of it.

What therefore will they regain? They should regain full understanding of the spiritual world. And the deed of Christ can only be grasped by self-aware human beings when they gain full understanding of Christ himself. The power of Christ certainly exists. Humankind did not bring it to earth for it came through Christ. Through Christ the possibility of karma entered humanity. But now human beings, as self-aware beings, must recognize the nature of Christ and his connection with the whole world. Only by this means can each person really act as an I. Following Christ's life on earth, what do we actually do if, rather than just allowing the power of Christ to work upon us unconsciously, rather than just being satisfied that Christ lived on earth and will redeem us—ensuring somehow that we progress—we undertake to perceive the real nature of Christ, *how* he descended, and to participate in Christ's deed through our own spirit. What is the significance of doing this?

Let us remind ourselves that we descended into the sensory world because luciferic spirits insinuated themselves into the human astral body, and that although this meant we could succumb to evil it also enabled us to achieve self-aware freedom. Lucifer dwells in the human being, and as it were fetched him down to the earth, enmeshing him in earthly existence. He did so by first leading earthwards the passions and desires present in the astral body so that Ahriman could then also attack us in the etheric body, in the mind soul. But then Christ appeared, and with him the power that can lead us upwards again into the world of spirit. And now, if we wish, we can perceive Christ! Now we can gather together all wisdom in order to recognize Christ. And what does this mean? Something of vast importance! When we perceive and acknowledge Christ, when we really allow ourselves to absorb the wisdom that tells us what he is, to penetrate this with understanding, then we redeem both ourselves and the luciferic beings through knowledge of Christ. If we are merely satisfied that Christ once lived on earth, we allow ourselves to be redeemed unconsciously! And then we would never help redeem the luciferic beings. These beings, who brought us freedom, also enable us to freely use this freedom to understand Christ. Then the luciferic spirits are purged and purified in the fire of Christianity, and the sin the luciferic spirits afflicted earth with is transformed from a sin into a boon, a benevolent deed. Freedom is achieved but is taken into the spiritual sphere as a deed of benevolence. That we are able to do this, are capable of perceiving and understanding Christ and that Lucifer is resurrected in a new form and can unite as the holy spirit with Christ is something Christ himself prophesied to those around him when he said, 'You can be illumined with the new spirit, with the holy spirit!'[66] This holy spirit is none other than the one through whom we can also come to understand the real nature of Christ's deed. Christ did not wish merely to work and act, but also desired to be understood. It is therefore integral to Christianity that the spirit who inspires us, the holy spirit, is sent to humankind.

Whitsun is spiritually connected with Easter, and cannot be seen apart from it. This holy spirit is none other than the resurrected luciferic spirit, reborn now in purer, higher glory—the spirit of independent, wisdom-imbued insight. Christ himself prophesied the advent of this spirit after him, and our further work must accord with it. What furthers this spirit? The world stream of spiritual science does so, when properly understood! What is this world stream? It is the wisdom of the spirit, which raises to full consciousness what would otherwise remain unconscious in Christianity.

Lucifer resurrected, and transformed into good, precedes Christ with the flaming torch. He bears Christ himself. He is the bearer of light, and Christ is the light. The name Lucifer means 'light-bearer'. That is precisely what the spiritual-scientific movement is to be, and what it signifies. And those who have understood that humanity's progress depends on understanding the great event of Golgotha are united, in the great guiding lodge of humanity, as the Masters of Wisdom and of the Harmony of Feelings.[67] And as long ago the tongues of fire descended upon the group of Apostles in a living, universal symbol, so the holy spirit sent by Christ himself holds sway as light over the lodge of the twelve. The thirteenth is the leader of this lodge. The holy spirit is the great teacher of those we refer to as the Masters of Wisdom and the Harmony of Feelings. They are therefore the ones through whom its voice and treasures of wisdom flow down to humanity on earth in one or another stream. The wisdom gathered together by the spiritual-scientific movement in order to understand the world and the spirits dwelling there flows from the holy spirit into the lodge of the twelve, and ultimately this is what will gradually lead humanity to self-aware, free insight into Christ and the event of Golgotha. Engaging with spiritual science thus means understanding that Christ sent the spirit into the world, and that spiritual science is intrinsic to true Christianity. People will increasingly come to realize this. And they will then see that in spiritual science they have a positive treasure for life. Spiritual science enables us to gradually become conscious of Christ as the spirit illuminating the world. And the consequence of this will be our human progress here on this globe, in the physical world, in terms of ethics, in terms of the will and in terms of the intellect. Passing through physical life, the world will become ever more spiritualized. Human beings will become better, stronger and wiser, and will wish to look ever more deeply into the deep ground and sources of existence. They will take with them as fruits what they accomplish and master here in this life of the senses, bring it with them into supersensible life and then bring it back with them again from supersensible life at each new incarnation.

In this way the earth will increasingly become an expression of its spirit, of the Christ spirit, and understanding for spiritual science will gradually arise from the world's foundations. People will come to see that spiritual science is a real, positive power. Today, in various ways, humanity is close to losing the spirit entirely. In a recent public lecture I highlighted the fear people feel of genetically transmitted diseases, of problematic inherited traits. This fear is part and parcel of our materialistic age. Yet is it enough to bask in the illusion that we can dismiss this fear? Certainly not. Someone who does not bother with the world of spirit, and does not imbue his soul with what can flow from the

spiritual-scientific movement, succumbs to what comes from the physical line of descent. Imbuing ourselves with what we can receive from
the spiritual stream of the science of the spirit is the only way to master
what descends through the line of inheritance, rendering it insignificant
and gaining victory over all the inhibiting powers that approach us from
the external world. We do not achieve mastery over the sensory world
by philosophizing it away, by endless debate, by stating that the spirit
exists, but instead by permeating ourselves with this spirit, really
absorbing it, really having the will to acquaint ourselves with all its
aspects and details. Then, also, people will become ever healthier within
the physical world through spiritual science, for this will itself become
the medicine which renders us hale and sound in the physical world.

The real power of spiritual science will become ever clearer if we
consider what we enter when we pass through the gate of death. This is
something very hard indeed for modern people to gain insight into.
Why, they wonder, should they bother about what happens in the
world of spirit? At death, they think, they'll be going there anyway and
that will be soon enough to see and hear what is there! You can hear
countless versions of this same, somewhat comfortable view: 'Why
bother with the spirit before I die—I'll find all that out when I get
there. Whether or not I'm preoccupied with it before I die won't alter
my relationship with the spiritual world!' But this is not so. Those who
think like this will find a dark, gloomy world after death. It will be like
finding it hard to discern or distinguish anything much of the worlds of
spirit described in my book in *Theosophy*. You see, it is only by connecting our soul and spirit with the world of spirit while we dwell here
in the physical world that we become able to perceive the spiritual
world. We prepare ourselves to see it while here. The world of spirit is
there, and the capacity to see it must be developed here on earth—for
otherwise you will be blind in the spiritual world.

Spiritual science gives you the power without which you cannot
consciously penetrate the spiritual world at all. If Christ had not
appeared in the physical world, human beings would sink down and
succumb to this world, would be unable to enter the world of spirit. But
now we can be raised through Christ into the spiritual world so that we
can become conscious there and perceive it. This also requires us to

know how to connect with what Christ sent, with the spirit, for otherwise we remain unconscious. We must acquire our immortality, for unconscious immortality is not yet immortality. Master Eckhart put this very beautifully when he said: 'What use to man to be a king, if knowing not he is this thing?'[68] By this he meant: What use is the spiritual world to us if we do not know what the world of spirit is? You can acquire the capacity to perceive the spiritual world only in the physical world. Let that give heart to those who ask why human beings ever descended to the physical world in the first place. The human being descended so that he can come to perceive the spiritual world here. He would remain blind to it if he had not descended to earth, acquiring here the self-aware nature with which he can return to the spiritual world, so that it lies open and radiant before him.

Spiritual science, therefore, is not merely a world-view but something without which the immortal part of us cannot know anything of the immortal worlds. It is a real power, and it flows as reality into our soul. As you sit here, engaging with and studying spiritual science, you not only gain knowledge but grow into being something that you would not otherwise become. That is the difference between spiritual science and other world-views. All other world-views relate to knowledge, while anthroposophy relates to human existence.

If we put things together in the right way, we will have to see it like this. Precisely in this light Christ, the spirit, and all of spiritual science appear intrinsically and inwardly connected. In the face of this living context, everything that can be said in superficial terms today—such as that a western esoteric school staunchly opposes an eastern one[69]—pales into insignificance. There are not two types of esotericism, nor any antagonism between western and eastern spiritual science. There is only *one* truth. And if someone asks us why, if eastern and western esotericism are one and the same, eastern schools do not acknowledge Christ, we can reply that it is not up to us to give an answer. We have no obligation to reply to this, for we acknowledge the full scope of eastern esotericism. If they ask us whether we acknowledge what eastern esotericism says about Brahma and Buddha, we will reply that we certainly do! We understand what is meant when eastern schools tell us that Buddha rose to his lofty eminence by a particular path. We do not negate a single one of all the

eastern truths and, in so far as they are positive, we fully acknowledge
each and every one. But should that deter us from acknowledging
something that exceeds their scope? Certainly not! We acknowledge
what eastern esotericism says, but this does not prevent us from also, at
the same time, acknowledging western truths.

People—supposedly learned scholars—disparage the view of orien-
talists that the Buddha succumbed through excess consumption of
pork.[70] But we can gain insight into the deeper meaning of this: that
the Buddha imparted too much esoteric wisdom to those around him at
the time, so that this satiation led to a kind of karma for him. And then
we can acknowledge this, can see that of course there is deeper esoteric
wisdom underlying the statements made by oriental esotericists. But if
someone tells us that it is beyond comprehension that John the Divine
received the book of the Apocalypse on Patmos, amidst thunder and
lightning,[71] we reply: All who know what this signifies also know it to
be true. We do not deny one truth, but nor can we accept denial of
another. It does not occur to us to contradict the statement that the
astral body of Buddha was preserved and later incorporated into
Shankaracharya.[72] But this cannot prevent us from teaching that the
astral body of Jesus of Nazareth was preserved, appearing in a certain
number of images or imprints incorporated into various figures who
worked to further Christianity—such as St Francis of Assisi or Elisabeth
of Thuringia. We do not deny a single truth of oriental esotericism; at
most we may refute what it negates in western esotericism. And so, if
people ask us why the eastern stream negates what we say, and why
opposition exists between eastern and western schools, we must refrain
from replying. It would only be up to us to answer if we had any dispute
with eastern esotericism ourselves. We don't! The person who denies or
negates something is the one obliged to answer such a question, not the
one who affirms and acknowledges. This is quite self-evident. And from
this perspective, over the next few weeks, you will be able to trace the
connection between spiritual science and the event of Golgotha, raising
into a higher sphere the whole mission and vocation of the world
movement for spiritual science through insight into the fact that this
spiritual science is the realization and enactment of the inspiration and
power which Christ named the spirit.

And so we see how powers work together in the world, how all that apparently resists and opposes humanity's progress later turns out to be of benefit, a boon. And likewise we see that in the post-Atlantean era, passing from one age to the next, the spirit who liberated human beings will reappear in a new form: the leading light-bearer Lucifer will be redeemed. For everything in world dispensation is good, and evil only prevails for a certain period. This is why we can only believe in never-ending evil if we confuse the temporal with the eternal. We will never understand the nature of evil unless we ascend from the temporal to the eternal realm.

LECTURE 17

BERLIN, 27 APRIL 1909

THIS winter we embarked on a whole series of spiritual-scientific reflections, all informed by the specific aim of gaining an ever more intimate understanding of the whole nature of the human being. We studied the great riddle of humankind from many different angles. Today's deliberations will focus on something very mundane. But perhaps precisely through engaging with mundane things we may discover how we can encounter the riddles of life at every turn, and how they can lead us into the world's depths if we grasp them fully and learn to master and handle them. You see, the loftiest spirit should not be sought in some unknown, far-off realm, for it manifests in the most everyday realities. We can seek the greatest in the least, the world in a grain of sand, if we know how to do so. In this cycle of winter lectures, therefore, I would like to incorporate a reflection on the ordinary, everyday theme of laughing and weeping as seen from a spiritual-scientific perspective.

Laughing and weeping are certainly very mundane aspects of human life. However, only spiritual science can give us insight into them, because it reveals the deepest core of human nature—which clearly distinguishes us from the other natural kingdoms on this globe. We stand head and shoulders above our fellow creatures on earth precisely because, of all of them, we have attained to the greatest degree of godliness, participating most intensely in the divine. For this reason, only knowledge and insight that raise themselves to the spirit can really fathom human nature. It is important to focus properly on laughing and weeping for a moment, for they alone can dispel the prejudice that tries to relate our nature far too closely to that of animals. There are schools of thought, of course, that accentuate our resemblance to animals—the high intelligence demonstrated in much animal behaviour, which can sometimes be more reliable than human reason. The spiritual scientist is not greatly surprised at this, for he knows that when an animal engages in intelligent activity this does not derive from the animal as an individual but from the group soul.[73] It is of course very difficult to explain the term 'group soul' in a way that renders it comprehensible or convincing to external observation, although this is by no means impossible. But we can bear in mind one thing in particular, which if our observations are wide-ranging enough can be externally verified: animals neither laugh nor cry. No doubt some people will claim that animals do cry and laugh. But this is to ignore the real nature of laughing and crying, for only by doing so can we ascribe it to animals. Anyone who practises true soul observation will know that the animal can howl at most but not cry, and only grin at most but not laugh. We need to be aware of this distinction—between howling and crying, and between grinning and laughing. In fact, to cast light on the real nature of laughing and crying, we have to look back in time to very important events.

You will recall from lectures I have given in various places, in Berlin too—especially the lecture on the temperaments[74]—that two streams need to be distinguished in human life. One comprises all human qualities and characteristics that we receive through inheritance, from our parents and ancestors, and can in turn be passed on genetically to our offspring. The other consists of qualities and characteristics we have by virtue of being born with an individuality. The individuality wraps itself in inherited characteristics only as though in a kind of shawl, whereas its intrinsic characteristics and qualities come from former lives on earth, from previous incarnations.

Basically therefore we are twofold in nature, inheriting one aspect of ourselves from our forefathers, while we bring the other with us from our past incarnations. Thus we distinguish the true core of our being that passes from one lifetime to another, from incarnation to incarnation, as opposed to all that clothes us, accruing around our intrinsic core of being and consisting of inherited characteristics. Before we are born, our true core of individuality, which passes from one incarnation to another, is certainly already connected with our physical being; and we should not think, therefore, that under normal circumstances our individuality could be exchanged after birth with any other. Prior to birth, the individuality is already connected with a particular human body.

But the point at which this core of being, this human individuality, can start to work upon us, shaping and configuring us, is another matter. Once the child is born, the individual core of being is already present as we saw. But prior to birth this core being cannot as yet bring to fruition or unfold the effects of what it acquired as capacities in the previous life or in all previous lives. It has to wait until after birth. And so we can say that before birth the causes of all inherited qualities and characteristics are actively working on us—the features we inherit from father, mother and other ancestors. As stated, our core being is present already in all this, but it cannot engage in the whole active complex until the child has actually been born.

Then, once the child has first seen the light of day, this individual core of his being begins to reconfigure the organism. Naturally I am speaking of ordinary circumstances—there are also exceptional instances where things are different. The core being transforms the brain and the other organs so that they can become its tools. This is why a child at birth bears more of the characteristics he receives through inheritance, while his individual qualities gradually work their way into the organism's general nature. If we wish to speak of the individual's work on the organism before birth, this would belong in a quite different domain. For example, we could in fact say that the individuality is already at work in choosing the parents. But this too is really a work undertaken from without. All work before birth can be seen as undertaken from without by our individual core of being, mediated for example by the mother and so on. But the direct work of this core being on the organism does not begin until the child has been born. And this is also why the intrinsically human quality, our individual nature, can only gradually come to expression after birth.

The child therefore initially has certain characteristics in common with animals—qualities, specifically, which find their expression in what we wish to talk about today in connection with laughing and weeping. In the first period after birth, the child cannot really laugh and cry. He will usually start to cry around 40 days after birth, and then also learn to smile. This is because what has survived from former lives now starts to be active, and from then on first sinks down into the body's interior and from there makes corporeal nature into its means of expression. It is precisely this that raises us above animals, for we cannot say that an individual soul passes on from one animal incarnation to the next. The animal is sustained by the group soul, and we cannot say that an animal's individual nature reincarnates again. Instead it returns to the group soul and becomes something that only lives on in this animal group soul. It is only in the human being that what is developed in one incarnation is then passed on into a new incarnation after the transition through devachan. In this new incarnation it gradually transforms the organism so that the latter is no longer merely an expression of the characteristics of its physical forefathers but instead comes to express individual dispositions, talents and so on.

Laughing and weeping are evoked specifically by the activity of the I within the organism of a being constituted as we are. Only a being bearing its I within it, whose I is therefore not a group I as in the animal but instead dwells within the organism, can laugh or cry. Laughing and crying are in fact nothing other than a subtle, intimate expression of I-hood within corporeality. What actually happens when a person cries? Crying can only happen if the I feels weak in some respect in relation to what surrounds it in the outer world. When the I does not inhabit the organism, and is thus not individual, a sense of feeling weak in relation to the environment cannot arise. As the possessor of an I entity, we experience a certain discord or disharmony in our relationship with our surroundings. And this sense of disharmony comes to expression in our attempt to defend ourselves, as though recreating balance. How do we recreate balance? This happens when our I causes the astral body to contract. We can put it like this: in the sadness expressed in crying, the I senses a certain disharmony with the outer world and seeks to compensate for this, to redress the balance, by inwardly contracting the astral body, as it were compressing its forces. This is the spiritual process that underlies weeping.

Let's take weeping as an expression of sadness or grief. In each individual instance we would have to study the particular nature and cause of this grief. It can for example express a sense of being bereft, of losing something we were previously united with. The harmonious relationship of our I to the outer world would exist if what we have lost were still present. Disharmony arises when we have lost something and the I feels forlorn. Now the I contracts the powers of its astral body, as it were compressing it, in order to defend itself against this sense of abandonment. This is the expression of a grief that leads to weeping. the I, the fourth aspect of our being, contracts and compresses the powers of the third aspect, the astral body.

What is laughter? It arises from the opposite process. The I allows the astral body to go slack in a sense, to let its powers broaden and expand. Whereas contraction invokes the weeping state, slackening and expanding of the astral body leads to laughter, as spiritual observation discovers. Whenever someone weeps, clairvoyant awareness ascertains a contraction, a compression of the astral body by the I. Whenever someone laughs, on the other hand, the I causes the astral body to expand, broaden and become more filled and rounded. Crying and laughing can only arise by virtue of an I active within us rather than working as a group I from without. Since the I is not yet really active at birth but gradually starts becoming so, and initially has not yet, as it were, taken up the reins that govern the organism from within, the child cannot cry or laugh at first. He only learns to do so as the I becomes master of the inner reins that are first active in the astral body. And since, in turn, everything spiritual in us finds its expression in our corporeality, the latter being only the physiognomy of the spirit, con-centrated spirit, these qualities that have now been described express themselves in bodily processes. And by making the following clear we learn to understand these bodily processes spiritually.

The animal has a group soul, which we can also call a group I, and this group I endows it with its distinctive form. Why does the animal have such a specific, inwardly enclosed form? Because this is impressed upon it from the astral world and because it must then largely preserve this form. Our human form, as we have often remarked, encompasses all other animal forms in a harmonious totality. But this whole, harmonious human form, our physical corporeality, has to be more inwardly mobile than animal corporeality. It must not be as rigid in form as the animal body. We can already see this in our mobile physiognomy. Just observe the relatively immobile physiognomy of the animal, its rigidity. And then look at the mobile human form with its changes of gesture, facial expression and so forth. Within the bounds assigned to us, you will see that we have a certain mobility, that we retain the capacity to some degree to determine our own form through the I indwelling us. It is not self-evident, other than perhaps in a metaphorical way, to speak of the individual expression of intelligence in the features of a dog or a parrot as being comparable to that of human beings. General intelligence, yes, but not individualized, since in the dog, parrot, lion or elephant, general characteristics predominate. Our individual character is inscribed in our faces. And we can observe how the particular, individual soul inscribes itself in human physiognomy, especially in the aspects of it that are mobile. We have retained this mobility through our capacity to endow ourselves with form from within. That we can shape and form ourselves in this way raises us above the other kingdoms of nature.

The moment our I alters the general relationship of forces in our astral body, this also comes to bodily expression in our physiognomy. Our usual facial expression, the normal muscle tone prevailing throughout the day, has to change when the I effects a change in the forces of the astral body. When the I lets the astral body go slack instead of maintaining the usual tone or tension, expands it, the latter will in turn work less strongly on the ether body and physical body; and this results in certain muscles, which maintain certain positions in the normal interplay of forces, adopting a different position. Therefore, if the I renders the astral body looser, slacker, in a certain expression of soul, particular muscles have to adopt a different tension from the one which usually prevails. Thus laughter is nothing other than the physical expression, the expression in our physiognomy, of this slackening of the astral body caused by the I itself. From within, through the I's influence, the astral body brings about the muscle positions that give us our ordinary expression. If this tone or tension is released by the astral body, the muscles relax and expand, and laughter comes to expression. Laughter is a direct expression of the I's inner action on the astral body.

When the astral body is compressed by the I under the influence of grief, this compression follows on into the physical body, leading to a secretion of tears, which in a sense are like the draining of blood under the influence of the compressed astral body. That is how these processes work. And this is why laughter and weeping can only be expressed by a being capable of incorporating the individual I, and through it acting from within. The individualized I is therefore initiated where a being is capable of either tensing or relaxing the powers of the astral body from within. Whenever we meet someone who smiles at us, or weeps before us, we see living evidence of the human being's higher stature compared with that of the animal. You see, the I works from without upon the animal's astral body, and for this reason all conditions of tension in the animal astral body can also only be caused from without. The animal cannot impress its inner life upon its outward form in the way we find this expressed in laughter and weeping.

There is a good deal more to discover about laughter and weeping, however, if we observe the breathing process in someone who laughs or cries. Here we can really fathom the depths of what is at work. Observe the breathing of a crying person, and you will find it consists largely of a long outbreath and short inbreath. The reverse is true of laughing, where a short outbreath corresponds to a long inbreath. The breathing process is therefore something which changes in us under the influence of the processes we have just described. You need only use a little imagination to see why this might be so.

In the process of crying the astral body is contracted and compressed by the I, and this leads to an expressing of the breath in a long outbreath. In laughter, the astral body goes looser or slacker, and this is like pumping the air out of an enclosed space, thinning and dispersing it, whereupon air will be drawn in. This causes the long inbreath when someone is laughing. In these changes in the breathing process we can see the I's activity within the astral body. The group I external to the animal is something we can rediscover in its inner action in ourselves in this remarkable expression affecting the breathing process and causing changes to it. Let us therefore examine for a moment the universal significance of this process.

In the animal we find a breathing process that is, you can say, governed and regulated from without and is not subject to the sway of the inner, individual I as we have described this today. What sustains the breathing process, governs it in fact, was named 'nephesh' in the esoteric lore of the Old Testament. In reality this is a term that designates the 'animal soul'. In other words, nephesh is the group I of animals. And in the Bible it is stated quite correctly that 'the Lord God ... breathed into his [man's] nostrils the nephesh[75]—the animal soul—and man became a living soul'. People frequently misunderstand this of course, since they are unable to read such profound texts in our time. They read them in a narrow, one-sided way. For instance, when the Bible states that God breathed the nephesh or animal soul into man, this does not mean that God created this soul at that moment, for it already existed. The text does not say the nephesh did not yet exist. It existed, outwardly. And what God did was to transpose into the inner nature of the human being something that had previously existed externally as the group soul. The key thing is for us to fathom the depths of such a phrase. Then we can ask what the consequence was of the transposition of the nephesh into the inner nature of the human being. This gave the human being his ascendency over animals, making it possible for him to unfold the inner activity of his I—to laugh and cry and thereby to experience joy and pain in a way that enables these to work upon him.

And here we come to the important effect of pain and joy in our lives. If we had no I within us, we could not inwardly experience pain and joy; instead they would pass us by without reality. But since we have an I in us, and can work upon our astral body and thus our whole corporeality from within outwards, pain and joy become powers that act upon us. The pain and joy we experience in one incarnation is something we integrate and incorporate, then carry over into a subsequent incarnation. It works creatively upon us. We can therefore say that pain and joy became creative powers of the universe at the moment we learned to cry and laugh—that is, at the moment our I was transposed into our inner nature. So here we have the ordinary, daily phenomenon of weeping and laughing. But we fail to understand it if we do not know how this relates to the core spiritual aspect of our being, what occurs there between the I and the astral body when we weep or laugh.

But what shapes and forms us is engaged in continuous development. The fact we can laugh or weep in a general way is due to the capacity of our I to work upon our astral body. That is certainly correct. But on the other hand, the human being's physical body and also ether body were in fact already predisposed to allow the I to work upon them within him when he entered upon his first earthly incarnation. The human being had the capacity for this. If one were to squeeze an individual I into a horse this I would feel most ill at ease there, since it would be unable to act at all, or find any expression for its individual I nature. Imagine an individual I in a horse. The individual I would try to work on the horse's astral body, contracting or expanding it and so forth. But when an astral body is connected with a physical body and an ether body, the physical and ether body present an terrible obstruction if they cannot adapt to the forms of the astral body. It is like knocking your head against a brick wall. The I within the horse's being would try to compress the astral body, but its physical and ether body would not oblige, and in consequence the horse would go mad because of the refusal of the ether and physical body to respond. The human being had to be predisposed for such activity from the outset. This could only happen by endowing him from the beginning with a physical body with the real capacity to be an instrument for an I, one that the I could gradually come to master. In consequence the following can also happen: the physical body and the ether body can be inwardly mobile, real I bearers as it were, but the I can remain very undeveloped, not yet exerting the right mastery over physical body and ether body. We can see this in the fact that physical body and ether body behave as a covering for the I without as yet being a full expression of it. This is the case with people who laugh or weep involuntarily, who bleat at every opportunity and do not have the laughter (risorius) muscles under their control. Such people show their higher human nature within their physical and etheric bodies, yet at the same time reveal that they have not so far brought their humanity under the control of the I. That's why bleating laughter can seem so unpleasant. It shows that a person is at a higher stage in something he can't help than in something he can already do something about. It always makes an especially dire impression when a being does not show himself equal to the sublimity given him from without.

Thus laughter and weeping are, in some respects, certainly an expression of human egohood, and this is already clear from the fact that they can only arise through the I indwelling the human being. Crying can be the expression of the most dire egoism, for all too frequently it is a kind of inner revelling. Someone who feels bereft contracts his astral body with his I, seeking to make himself inwardly strong because he feels outwardly weak. And he feels this inner strength through being able to do something—that is, produce tears. And a certain sense of satisfaction is always connected with producing tears, whether we acknowledge this or not. Just as a kind of satisfaction is evoked in other circumstances when someone smashes a chair to pieces, so there is often nothing other than inner revelling involved in this generating of tears, a revelling in the mask of tears, even if we are not aware of this.

That laughter is in some way an expression of the I, of egohood can become clear from the fact that, if you really trace its origin, laughter must always be ascribed to a person feeling superior to his surroundings and what is happening there. Why do people laugh? It is always when they feel superior to what they observe. You can always discover the truth of this. Whether you laugh at yourself or someone else, basically your I feels superior to something. And in this sense of superiority the I expands the powers of its astral body, becomes broader, puffs itself up. This is what really underlies laughter. This is why laughing can be so good for you, and we should not condemn in an abstract way all egoity, all puffing up of oneself. Laughter can be very healthy when it strengthens our sense of ourselves in a justified way, leading us beyond ourselves. If you see something in your surroundings, in yourself and others, that is complete nonsense, your laughter elevates you above the nonsense going on there. It must sometimes happen that we rise above something in our surroundings; and the I expresses this by expanding the astral body.

If you relate the breathing process to the saying that God breathed the nephesh into the human being so that he became a living soul, you will also sense the connection here with laughing and weeping, for you know that the breathing process itself alters when we weep or laugh. We have thus shown how the most mundane occurrences can really only be understood when we approach them from a spiritual perspective. We can only understand the real nature of weeping and laughter through insight into the connection between the four aspects or levels of the human being. Just consider that in times when clairvoyant traditions still existed to some degree, along with a capacity to visualize the gods through true imaginative perception, the gods were depicted as blithe and jocund beings whose chief attribute, really, was jocularity and laughter. Nor was it for nothing that weeping and the gnashing of teeth were assigned to realms of universal existence in which an excessive egohood primarily held sway. Why? Because laughter signifies a raising of oneself, a leading of the I beyond its surroundings, and thus the victory of what is higher over what is lower, whereas weeping signifies cowering, withdrawing from the external, a sense of the ego growing smaller and feeling bereft, a retreat into oneself. In human life, grief is poignant and stirring because we know that it will and must be overcome, but in the world in which sadness and grief can no longer be overcome they do not appear poignant but hopeless. There they appear as the expression of damnation, of being cast out into the darkness.

When we consider the larger context of how the work of the I upon itself informs and is expressed in the human being, this can give rise to powerful feelings to which we must pay close attention and which we must pursue into their intimate configurations. We will then have grasped a good deal of what we encounter through the ages of evolution. We need an awareness of a spiritual world behind the physical, and of the fact that what arises in human life as the fluctuating phenomena of laughter and weeping appears, separately from us, as the bright blitheness of the heavens on the one hand and the dark, bitter grief of hell on the other. These two realms underlie our middle or mediating world, and we must see how this world draws its powers from both these other realms.

There are a good many other aspects of human nature which we will study, but this theme of laughing and crying is, I would say, one of the most intimate things we can learn about the human being, even though they are such ordinary, everyday occurrences. The animal does not laugh or weep because it does not have within it the divine spark that we bear in our I. When a child begins to smile and cry, those able to read the great script of nature will see in this a sign of the divine nature indwelling the human being. When someone laughs, a god acts within him, seeking to raise him above all that is lower—for smiling and laughter is elevation. And when someone weeps this is, on the other hand, a divine warning that this I might lose itself if it does not strengthen itself against all weakening and sense of being bereft. The god within us admonishes the soul in laughter and weeping. This is why someone who understands life will be overcome by something like deep annoyance when he sees someone crying unnecessarily. Unnecessary weeping shows that instead of living and feeling in sympathy with our surroundings there is too much voluptuous enjoyment of inhabiting one's own I. But the same insightful person will likewise experience an acerbic feeling when he witnesses an otherwise healthy elevation of the I over its surroundings in laughter, as an end in itself, as generalized laughter and smirking disparagement. For then this person says: If the I does not take with it everything it can draw out of its surroundings, if it does not wish to live in responsive engagement with these surroundings but instead unjustifiably elevates its I over them, this I nature will not have the necessary gravity, upward gravity, that can be found only by drawing from the environment everything that can be drawn from it to nurture the development of the I. And then the I will fall back, will be unable to raise itself. It is precisely the right balance between pain and joy that can contribute so hugely to human development. If pain and joy in our surroundings are justified, do not lie only within us, and if between pain and joy the I continually seeks to establish the right relationship to its surroundings then pain and joy can become proper developmental factors for us.

This is why great poets frequently find such beautiful words for the pain and joy that are not rooted in either the I's sense of superiority or its inward compression, but whose cause lies in the externally disrupted balance of the relationship between the I and its surroundings—as the only way of understanding why someone may laugh or cry. We can understand this because we see how the relationship between I and external world is disrupted in and by the external world. So we must laugh or cry whereas—if the cause lies only within someone—we cannot understand what makes him laugh or cry, since then it is always unjustified egoism. That is why we find it so beautiful when Homer says of Andromache, who suffers from a double anxiety for both her husband and her infant: 'She wept laughingly!'[76] That is a wonderful phrase for something we can see as normal in weeping. She does not laugh or cry for her own sake. She has the right relationship to her surroundings when troubled both for her husband on the one hand and her child on the other. And here, as they hold the balance with each other, we have the right relationship between laughter and tears: weeping smilingly— laughing through tears. This is also often something expressed by the young child whose I is not yet so inwardly hardened as later in the adult, so that he can still laugh as he weeps and weep as he laughs. And we find it again in a wise person: someone who has overcome himself sufficiently to look beyond himself to discover why he laughs and weeps, discovering this in the world around him. Again, such a person can weep laughingly and laugh weepingly. Yes, indeed, in what we often fail to notice in ordinary daily life, the spirit comes to full expression. Laughing and weeping are something that we can, in the most lofty sense, see as a divine physiognomy within us.

LECTURE 18

TODAY we will try to enlarge a little on the manifold esoteric realities and outlooks that we have elaborated this winter. It has often been emphasized that what we call spiritual science should engage in human life, and can become living actions and deeds. Today, though, let us add a little to our picture of the great evolutionary processes at work in the universe, as these come to expression in the human being. And first of all let me guide you towards a fact which, if you regard it in the right way, can be very helpful in explaining the nature of world evolution.

Consider for a moment the purely external difference between human and animal development. A single word suffices to evoke the difference between the concept of animal development and that of humans. This is the word 'education'. Education in the proper sense of the word cannot apply to animals. Of course we can use dressage and training to induce animals to behave in certain ways that deviate from their natural instincts—from what they possess as predisposition and comes to natural expression. But one must really be a very keen dog lover indeed to deny the radical difference between human education and what can be undertaken with an animal. In fact we need only recall an important insight provided by our anthroposophical world-view to find a deeper basis for this initially superficial observation.

We know that human beings develop gradually in a very complex way. We have repeatedly emphasized how, during the first seven years of life up to the change of teeth, the child's development unfolds in a way quite different from the next seven years, up to the age of 14, and

then in a different way again from the age of 14 through to 21. I just
mention this in passing since you're aware of it. A spiritual-scientific
view of things shows us that the human being is 'born' several times as
he develops.

We are born into the physical world when we leave the mother's
body, shedding the physical mother envelope. But having done so, we
know that we are still enclosed in another, a second, etheric mother
envelope. As he grows towards the age of seven, what we call the child's
etheric body is surrounded on all sides by external ether streams
belonging to the surrounding environment, in the same way that the
physical body is surrounded by the physical mother envelope until birth.
This second, etheric envelope is shed at second dentition, and then the
ether body is born around the seventh year. At this point, however, the
astral body is still enclosed in the astral envelope, which is shed at
puberty. After this, the human astral body develops freely until the
twenty-first or twenty-second year, when the true I is really first born.
Only at this point does a person awaken to full inner intensity, when
what has developed as I through his various former incarnations first
works its way out and emerges from within.

A quite singular fact becomes apparent here to clairvoyant consciousness. If you observe a young child for a few weeks, or perhaps
months, you will see that his head is surrounded by etheric and astral
streams and forces. These etheric-astral streams and forces however
become gradually less apparent and fade after a while. What is actually
happening here? In fact you can work out what is happening without
clairvoyant faculties, though clairvoyance confirms what I am going to
say. The human brain directly after birth is not the same as it is later,
after a few weeks or months. While the baby already perceives the outer
world, his brain does not as yet provide an instrument for combining
external impressions in a particular way. Separate connecting nerves
running from one part of the brain to another only develop after birth.
These connective nerves, by means of which we gradually learn to link
in thought what we see outside us, only slowly form after the child has
been born. Let's say that a child hears a bell ring, and also sees it ringing,
but he will not immediately connect the auditory and visual impression
with the idea: It is that bell which is ringing. He only gradually learns to

do so, since the part of the brain that is the instrument for perceiving tones and the part responsible for visual perception only gradually become connected. Only then can the child appraise a situation properly and say that what he sees is also what is making the sound.

Thus connecting links are formed in the brain, and the forces that enable these links to emerge and form can be seen clairvoyantly in the first few weeks as extra enveloping layers around the brain. But what envelops the brain at this point subsequently enters and lives within it. It no longer works from without but within the brain itself. What works from without in the first few weeks of child development could not work further on the growing child's whole development if it were not protected by the various enveloping layers. You see, when what I have just described as working from without enters the brain and is within it, it continues to develop first under the protecting envelope of the ether body and then of the astral body. Only around the age of 21 does what has worked from without until then now become active from within. What was initially outside the child in the first moments of life, then slipped inside, does not work unprotected—without any envelope at all—until the age of 19 to 21. At that point it becomes free and develops the intensity I spoke of.

Now let us consider for a moment this gradual process of human development. Let us compare it with the development of the plant. We know that the plant here in the physical world, where we initially encounter it, only has a physical and ether body, and that its astral body is outside and surrounds it. Within itself it has only a physical and ether body. The plant emerges from the seed, forms its physical body and gradually its etheric body also arises. But the plant only has this ether body. Now we saw that the human ether body still has its astral body around it up to puberty, and that the astral body is only really born then. By contrast the plant, after reaching sexual maturation, cannot give birth to an astral body of this kind since it does not possess one. The necessary consequence of this is that at sexual maturation the plant now has nothing more that needs to be developed. It has fulfilled its task in the physical world once sexual maturation is achieved, and dies after fertilization.

In some lower animals you can see something similar; in them, unlike higher animals, the astral body is really not yet drawn right down into the physical body. Lower animals are distinguished precisely by the fact that the astral body is not yet within the physical body. Take the mayfly as an example; it develops, lives until fertilization, is fertilized and then dies. Why? Because it is a creature whose astral body, as in the plant, is largely outside it and can therefore develop nothing further once sexual maturation has occurred.

In a certain respect, humans, animals and plants develop in similar ways until sexual maturity. But the plant then has no further developmental task in the physical world and dies after sexual maturation. The animal has an astral body within it but no I. After sexual maturity therefore, it still has a certain reserve of developmental potential. The astral body becomes free, and for as long as it goes on freely developing, for as long as it retains developmental potential, the animal's further development will continue after sexual maturity. Now the animal's astral body in the physical world has no I within it. The animal's I is a group I, always comprising a whole group and existing in the astral world as group I. This group I in the astral world has quite different developmental possibilities than does the animal here in the physical world. But the astral body that the animal possesses has very limited scope for development. At birth already the animal bears this developmental potential within it. The lion has something that comes to expression in its astral body as a sum of drives, instincts and passions. And these drives, desires and passions *can* come to expression in its astral body. This all lives until the point at which an I could be born—but an I is not present, existing instead on the astral plane. Therefore when the animal has arrived at the level of a human being approaching the age of 21, its developmental potential has been exhausted.

The actual length of time an animal lives naturally varies depending on circumstances—not all animals live to be 21. But human beings up to the age of 21, when the I is born, share in what is intrinsically animal development up to that point. This does not of course mean that human development up to the age of 21 is animal in nature. It is not, for what becomes free at 21 is already within us from the very beginning, from conception, and is now freed. The human being is not animal in nature because something exists in him from the beginning which becomes free from the age of 21. This I works in him from the outset, albeit in unfree form. And it is this I in fact that can be educated. It is this I, along with what it elaborates and develops through the astral, etheric and physical body, that passes from incarnation to incarnation. If nothing new were added to this I at each new incarnation, we would be unable, at our physical death, to take with us anything from our past life between birth and death. And if we could not do so, in our subsequent life we would find ourselves on exactly the same level as in the preceding one. We continually enrich our I by virtue of the fact that we undergo a process of development during our lifetime, acquiring and absorbing things that the animal cannot because its developmental potential is circumscribed. This means that we can rise ever higher from incarnation to incarnation. And because we bear an I within us that is not born until we are 21, but which is at work in us prior to that, we can be educated and can make of ourselves something other than we were predisposed or predetermined to be from the beginning. The lion brings its lion nature with it and gives expression to it. The human being brings not only his generally human attributes as member of a species but also what he acquired as I in his last incarnation. And this can be transformed ever more through education and life so that it is endowed with a new impetus when we pass through the gate of death and must then prepare ourselves for a new incarnation. It is this we must keep in mind: that we absorb new developmental factors and continually enhance our potential.

But now let us ask what happens really when we outwardly enhance ourselves through developmental factors of this kind. Here we must first try to grasp three very important concepts which are hard to comprehend. We have been working together in these branch meetings for many years now, and so no doubt it will be possible to progress to somewhat more advanced concepts. To formulate the three concepts, first consider a fully grown plant—if you like a lily of the valley. There you have the plant before you in a particular form. You could equally well have it before you in a different form, though, as a small seed. If you look at this small seed form in front of you, you can become aware that it contains everything that will later become visible as root, stem, leaves and flowers. So first I have the flower before me as a seed, and then also as a full-grown plant. Yet the seed could not lie here in front of me if it had not been created by a previous lily of the valley. But for clairvoyant consciousness something else is also true. When clairvoyant consciousness observes the full-grown lily of the valley, it sees its physical form permeated by an ether body, a kind of body of streaming light penetrating it from top to bottom. In the case of the lily of the valley, however, the ether body does not extend very far beyond the physical body of the plant and is not much different from it. But if you take the lily of the valley's small seed, while the physical seed is small, you will find that a wondrous ether body incorporates itself into this seed in a radiant circular form. The seed itself sits at one end of the ether body similar to the way a comet's nucleus relates to its tail. The physical seed is in fact only a concentrated point in the light or ether body of the lily of the valley.

Someone who studies things from a spiritual-scientific perspective will find that he has before him in the fully-grown lily of the valley an unfolding of what was first hidden. In relation to the seed before him, where the physical is very small and only the spiritual aspect is large, he can say that the true being of the lily of the valley is wrapped inside the physical seed. Thus in observing the lily of the valley we must distinguish two different conditions: one in which the lily of the valley's whole being is involuted, infolded, wrapped up in the seed; and another in which this initial state unfolds and passes into evolution as the plant grows. But then the lily of the valley's whole being slips in turn into the new, growing seed. This unfolding and infolding alternate in the developmental sequences of a plant's being. During unfolding or evolution, the spiritual fades increasingly while the physical aspect becomes hugely pronounced; then during infolding or involution, the physical will increasingly vanish while the spiritual aspect grows ever more potent.

In a sense we can say that evolution and involution alternate in us too, but in a still more palpable way. In a human being between birth and death, a physical body and an ether body unite in physical existence, as does the spiritual element in a certain way. As earthly human beings we have 'unfolded'. But when you clairvoyantly observe a human soul pass through the gate of death, he does not leave behind in physical life even as much as a lily of the valley seed. The physical vanishes so utterly that you no longer see it, and everything is infolded into the realm of spirit. The soul now passes through devachan, and is infolded in relation to his earthly being. In relation to our earthly being we have evolution, unfolding between birth and death, and involution, infolding, between death and a new birth. But there is an enormous difference between a person and a plant. In relation to the plant we can speak of evolution and involution, but in the case of a human being there is a third thing to consider as well. Without this third thing we could not fully encompass a human being's whole development. Since the plant always passes through involution and evolution, every new plant repeats the old one, is exactly the same as it. The nature of the lily of the valley always infolds itself into the seed and unfolds again. What happens in the case of the human being?

We have just acknowledged that during life between birth and death we take up new elements of developmental potential and enhance ourselves. The human being thus differs from the plant. A person's next earthly unfolding is not mere repetition of his preceding one, but allows enhancement of his existence. What we absorb or integrate between birth and death we also infold into what previously existed, and therefore instead of mere repetition what subsequently unfolds appears at a higher level. Where does what we absorb and integrate actually come from? What does it mean to acquire, absorb and integrate a new element? Please pay very careful attention here—we are approaching a most important and most difficult concept. And there is good reason why I am saying this in one of our last sessions for you will have the whole summer to reflect on it. We should reflect on such concepts for months and years for then we gradually engage with the whole profundity they contain. Where does what is continually integrated into our being originate? Let us try to make this clear through a simple example.

Assume there is someone in front of you who is looking at two others. Now bring together everything that belongs to evolution, to unfolding. We can say of the person who stands before us and observes the other two that he has passed through former incarnations, has unfolded what these past lives implanted in him. This is true also of the other two who stand facing him. But now assume that the first person takes pleasure in the way the two others are standing beside each other—the sight of these particular two people standing next to each other pleases him. Someone else might well not experience this pleasure that the first experiences in seeing these two. The pleasure he feels has nothing to do with the developmental potential of the two others, for their capacity to give pleasure to the first by standing next to each other is not something they have acquired. It is something else entirely and is due solely to the fact that *he* is the one standing there before them. So here you have a person developing an inward feeling of pleasure due to the fact that those two are standing there before him. This feeling is not brought about by anything to do with evolution, with unfolding. There are things in the world which arise solely through the way realities are juxtaposed. It is not a matter of the two people being linked through karma. So now let us consider this pleasure which the one feels through having the other two standing there side by side.

Take another example. Someone is standing at a certain place and turns his gaze towards a particular constellation in the heavens. If he were standing five steps further on he would see something different. The sight awakens a sense of pleasure in him, one that is new and original. Thus we experience a sum of realities that are entirely new and are not determined by our former development. Everything relating to the lily of the valley lies in its earlier development. But this is not true of the ways in which our surroundings act upon our soul. There are all sorts of factors that have nothing to do with a former developmental process, but which arise when certain circumstances bring us into contact with the outer world. By experiencing this pleasure, it becomes something within us, however, and gives rise in our soul to something that is not predetermined by anything that has gone before. Something arises from nothing. Such creative beginnings from nothing continually arise in the human soul. These are soul experiences which we do not experience through facts or realities but through interrelationships that we ourselves elaborate between facts. It is important to distinguish between experiences we acquire from realities, or from interrelationships between realities.

Life really falls into two aspects that interweave without clear boundaries: experiences strictly determined by former causes, by karma, and those not karmically caused that enter fresh and new into our field of vision. For example, there are whole areas of human life that fall into this latter category. Imagine you get news that someone has stolen something. Of course whatever may have happened is determined by certain karmic factors. But assume you have just got wind of the theft yet do not know the person who committed it. In objective reality it has been committed by a quite specific person whom, however, you do not know. The thief does not approach you to say, 'Please lock me up, I was the one who did it.' No, you have to construe the facts from all sorts of hints in a way that may tell you who the thief might be. The ideas you formulate in the process have nothing to do with the objective facts. They are dependent on quite different things, including how clever you are or not. The train of thought you formulate does not have to lead to the actual thief either, but is a process that unfolds only within you, to complement external reality. Basically all logic is something that is added to reality, as are all aesthetic judgements. So we continually enhance and enrich our lives through things that are not rooted in previous causes but that we experience by relating ourselves in one way or another to reality.

If we now take a quick journey through the whole of human life and recall how it evolved through the stages of old Saturn, old Sun and old Moon to our present Earth evolution, we find that it was not yet possible on Saturn for the human being to form such interconnections. Necessity alone prevailed. The same was true on old Sun and old Moon; and the way humans were on old Moon is how things still are for animals today. The animal's experience is determined by preceding causes. Only the human being has entirely new, not previously determined experiences. This is why only humans can be educated in the true sense of the word. The human being alone keeps adding something new to what is karmically determined. Only on earth do we acquire the capacity to add something new. On old Moon we had not yet evolved far enough to be able to add anything new to our original disposition and potential. Although we were not animals then either, we stood at the level of animal evolution. We were determined by outer causation in whatever we undertook. But we still are today to a certain degree, for free experiences only slowly work their way into us, doing so all the more as we raise ourselves to higher levels of evolution.

Consider Raphael's paintings, and imagine a dog regarding them. It will see what is objectively there, whatever arises from them in so far as they are sensory objects. But now imagine a human being looking at these pictures. He will see something quite different in them—something he can only conceive by having passed through former incarnations and evolved. And now take a brilliant person, a genius, someone like Goethe; he sees more still, understands the full significance of these paintings, and why one is painted in one way, another in another. The more highly evolved we become, the more we perceive. Thus the more we have previously enhanced our soul, the more we complement what we see with these kinds of interrelationships experienced in our soul. And these become soul possessions, taking root in our soul. But all this has only become possible for humanity since the beginning of Earth evolution. The following occurs however.

As time progresses human beings continue to evolve. We know that the Earth stage will be followed by Jupiter, Venus and Vulcan. During this process of evolution, the sum of experiences we have undergone over and above preceding causes will continually increase, and our inner life will grow ever richer. What we have brought with us from old causes, from Saturn, Sun and Moon evolution, will become ever less significant. We will evolve beyond former causation and cast it off. And when we have reached the planetary stage of Vulcan, we will have shed everything we absorbed and incorporated during Saturn, Sun and Moon evolution. We will have cast all this off.

Now we come to a difficult idea that I will try to explain with a metaphor. Picture yourself sitting in a car that you have either inherited or has been given to you. You take a trip in this car, but one wheel has something wrong with it, and you replace the faulty wheel with a new one. So then you have the old car with one new wheel. Now let's also assume that a second wheel develops a fault after a while, so that you have to change this one too. You're now driving in the old car with two new wheels. This repeats itself until you have replaced the third and fourth wheel, then other parts of the car. It's easy to imagine that at some point the car you are driving will no longer contain anything at all of the old one. You no longer have anything left of what you inherited or were given. You sit there in the car but really it is a new vehicle. Now transpose this to human evolution. During the Saturn times we received the germ of our physical body, and gradually developed it; then during Sun evolution we acquired the ether body, during the Moon stage the astral body, and during Earth evolution the I. Gradually we develop and elaborate these. But within the I we increasingly develop new experiences, casting off what we inherited, what we were endowed with during Saturn, Sun and Moon stages. And a time will come—the Venus period of evolution—when we will have shed all that the gods gave us during Moon, Sun, Saturn and the first half of Earth evolution. We will have cast all this off just as the various parts of the car were replaced in our metaphor. And we gradually replace all this with what we absorb from conditions that did not previously exist. We will not be able to arrive on Venus and maintain that everything we acquired through Saturn, Sun, Moon and Earth evolution is still there in us, for we will have shed all of this. And at the end of our evolution we will bear in us only what we ourselves have elaborated, have created out of nothing, and not what was bestowed on us.

This then is the third aspect that is added to evolution and involution—creation out of nothing. Unfolding, infolding and creation out of nothing: this is what we must call to mind if we wish to grasp the whole grandeur and majesty of human evolution. And so we can understand how the gods first gave us the vehicle of our three bodies, how they gradually built this vehicle and then gave us the capacity to slowly master and overcome it so that we might cast it off bit by bit. In this process the gods wish gradually to make us in their image, as a being that can say to itself, 'I was given the predisposition to become what I should, but I have created a whole new entity out of these rudiments.'

Great, elevated spirits previously evolved what we look forward to as a great, wonderful ideal—not only of self-awareness but awareness of our self-creation. And what we will only experience in a far-distant future is being evolved now by certain spirits that once participated in our evolution. During Saturn evolution, as we have seen, the Thrones poured out what we call the substance of humanity, into which the Spirits of Personality in turn poured what we can call the powers of personality. But these Spirits of Personality, who were at that time powerful enough to pour their personality character into this substance poured out by the Thrones, have since ascended ever higher. Today they have attained the stage of no longer needing physical substance for their further evolution. On Saturn they needed physical Saturn substance to be able to live at all—and this substance was at the same time the germ of human substance. On old Sun they needed etheric substance which flowed out to become the human ether body; on old Moon they needed astral substance, and here in Earth evolution they need our I. But henceforth they will need what this I itself elaborates when we create something new out of pure conditions—something that is no longer physical, ether and astral body as such, and no longer I, but instead proceeds from the I and is produced by it. The Spirits of Personality will use this and are already doing so in order to live within it. On Saturn they lived in what is today our physical body, on Sun in what is our ether body and on Moon in what is now our astral body. Since the middle of Atlantean times, they have begun to live in what human beings can bring forth as higher reality from their I.

What kinds of higher reality do people produce from their I? There are three. First, what we call lawful thinking, our logical thinking. This is something we bring towards things. If we do not merely look out into the external world, do not merely observe—not just running after the thief to find him—but allow the lawfulness inherent in our observation to dawn on us, we live in logic, true logic. Then we formulate thoughts that have nothing directly to do with the thief and yet they may catch up with him. This logic is something that comes from us, is added by us to complement things. In giving ourselves to this true logic, the I is creative over and above itself.

Secondly the I is creative over and above itself when it finds pleasure and displeasure in things that are beautiful, elevated, humorous, funny—in short, in things that human beings themselves produce. Let us say you see something out in the world that strikes you as stupid and you laugh at it. The fact of your laughter itself is not in the least dependent on your karma. A dull-witted person might view the same thing you are laughing at as very astute. Your response arises from the singular outlook that you yourself have. Or let us say that you see a hero who is being assaulted by the world, initially managing to hold his own but perishing tragically in the end. What you observe is determined by karma, but the sense of tragedy you yourself feel as you witness it is quite new.

Lawfulness or necessity in thinking is the first aspect, pleasure and displeasure the second. The third is the way in which you feel urged to act under the sway of circumstances. This too is not solely karmically determined but arises from your relationship to the matter in hand. Let us assume that two people have a relationship in which karma determines that they have something to make amends for together. At the same time, though, the development of one of them is more advanced than that of the other. The more advanced person will make amends while the other postpones this for later, doing so at a later time. One of the two will develop goodness of heart while the other does not participate in such feelings. Here something new starts to develop. You must not regard everything as determined, but it depends on whether or not we allow our actions to be governed by the laws of justice and equity. Ever new things arise in our morality, in the way we fulfil our obligations and in our moral judgement. In our moral judgement, especially, lies the third aspect by means of which we raise ourselves beyond ourselves, by means of which the I increasingly makes progress. The I creatively integrates this into our earthly world, and what is incorporated in this way does not fade again. What human beings creatively infuse into the earth from epoch to epoch, from age to age, as the results of logical thinking, aesthetic judgement and the fulfilment of duties forms an ongoing stream and provides the matter and substance in which the Spirits of Personality embed themselves at their present stage of evolution.

Thus you live your life and develop yourself. And as you do so, the Spirits of Personality look down upon you and continually ask you whether you are giving them something they can use for their own evolution. In developing thought content, riches of thought, in attempting to refine and enhance our aesthetic judgement and fulfil our obligations over and above what arises from karma, in giving nourishment to the Spirits of Personality through these offerings, we help the corpus of these Spirits of Personality to become more concentrated.

What do these Spirits of Personality embody? Something that human beings regard as abstract: the *zeitgeist*, the spirit of diverse epochs. Someone who takes the stance of spiritual science regards this spirit of the time as a real being. The Time Spirits, who are none other than the Spirits of Personality, process through the ages. If we look back to ancient times, to Indian, Persian, Chaldean-Babylonian and Graeco-Roman culture, and through to our own time, we find that, quite apart from the diverse nations and other human differences, the presiding Time Spirit always changes. Five thousand years ago people thought and felt differently to now, and three thousand years ago differently again. The Spirits of Time, or the Spirits of Personality are what change, if we use terms drawn from spiritual science. These Spirits of Personality undergo an evolution in the supersensible realm, in the same way that the human race evolves in the sensory domain. But what we, the human race, unfold into the supersensible realm is food and drink for these Spirits of Personality—they relish it. If human beings lived without developing a rich life of thinking, without pleasure or displeasure, without a sense of duty that goes beyond merely karmic dictates, the Spirits of Personality would have nothing to 'eat' and would grow gaunt. Thus our life stands in relation to such beings, who invisibly interweave with our life, live through and in it.

I said that we add something new to evolution, as it were creating out of nothing to complement involution and evolution, but that we could not create anything out of nothing if we had not first received the causes into which we placed ourselves as in a vehicle. This vehicle was given us during Saturn evolution; piece by piece we throw it overboard and develop into the future. But we must first have received the foundation to do so, and if the gods had not first created this foundation for us we could not have created anything out of nothing. It is due to these strong foundations that the interrelationships we inhabit can act upon us and be truly fruitful for our further development. What, in fact, has become possible through our capacity to create something new from what is given, to make the interrelationships in which we are embedded into a foundation for new things that we ourselves create, to think things that go beyond the actual reality we experience around us, to feel more than stands purely objectively before us? What has become possible through our capacity to act over and above the dictates of karma and to live with a sense of obligation towards truth, equity and goodness of heart?

The human capacity to think logically, to develop necessity and lawfulness in thinking, also gave rise to the possibility of error. The human capacity to take pleasure in beauty also made it possible to engraft what is ugly or sullied upon world evolution. Our capacity to develop and embrace a concept of duty over and above mere karma also created the potential for evil, for rejecting our obligations. Precisely through our potential for creating more than is bestowed on us by circumstances, to be creative within them, we have been transposed into a world in which we can also create and weave our spiritual substance in a way that renders it full of error, ugliness and evil. And more than just making it possible for human beings to create at all out of their circumstances, their interrelationships, it had to be made possible for them gradually to create truth and beauty from given conditions by their striving and struggling: gradually to create the virtues that can really enable us to progress in evolution.

In Christian esotericism, creating something new from given conditions is called 'creating in the spirit', while creation drawn from right (or true), beautiful and virtuous conditions is called the 'holy spirit'. The holy spirit inspires us when we are able to create truth, beauty and goodness out of nothing. But the foundation necessary for us to become capable of creating in accord with this holy spirit first had to be bestowed on us, as for all creation, out of nothing. This foundation was given us through Christ's entry into our evolution. When we were able to experience the Christ event on earth, we became able to ascend to creation in the holy spirit. It is therefore Christ himself who creates the fullest, deepest foundation. If we can stand upon the ground of the Christ experience so that Christ becomes the vehicle into which we enter to evolve further, Christ sends us the holy spirit and we become able to create what is right, beautiful and good in harmony with the further course of evolution.

Thus, in a sense as ultimate conclusion of what was imprinted into us through Saturn, Sun and Moon evolution, we see how the Christ event on earth endowed us with the highest aspect, enabling us to work our way into a future perspective and increasingly to create something new over and above given circumstances—drawing not on what exists here or there as a given, but instead arises from how we relate to the facts of our environment, which is the holy spirit in the broadest sense. That in turn is an aspect of Christian esotericism. Christian esotericism is connected with the profoundest idea we can have of all evolution, with the idea of creating out of nothing.

This is why no true theory of development can ever dispense with the idea of creation out of nothing. If only unfolding and infolding obtained, there would be eternal repetition as we see in the plant, and on Vulcan there would only exist what commenced on Saturn. But unfolding and infolding are complemented by creation out of nothing at the midpoint of our development. After Saturn, Sun and Moon stages pass away, Christ descends to earth as the great enriching, enhancing element that will lead to something entirely new appearing on Vulcan, something that did not exist on Saturn. Those who speak only of unfolding and infolding regard development in terms of the endless recurring of everything, an endlessly repeating cycle. Such cycles, though, can never properly explain the evolution of the universe. Only when we add to unfolding and infolding development this creation out of nothing, which incorporates something new into given conditions, do we really start to understand the world.

Lower entities reveal at most a hint of what we can call creation out of nothing. A lily of the valley repeatedly gives rise to more lilies of the valley. At most a gardener may externally add something to the lily of the valley that it would never otherwise have developed by itself. Then the plant could be called a creation out of nothing. We human beings, though, are capable of incorporating this creation out of nothing into ourselves. We only become capable of this, though, by raising ourselves to this freedom of self-creation through the freest deed we look upon as our example and paradigm. What freest deed is this? It is that the wise, creating Word of our solar system took the inner resolve to enter a human body and participate in the earth's evolution, to enact a deed that lay in no preceding karma. When Christ resolved to enter a human body, he was not compelled to this by any preceding karma but took it upon himself as a free deed. This was founded solely on a prefiguring vision of the future evolution of humanity, which had never previously existed but first arose in him as a prefiguring thought created out of nothing. This is a difficult idea, but Christian esotericism will never be able to ignore it, and everything depends on our capacity to add the idea of creation out of nothing to that of unfolding and infolding development and evolution.

If we are able to do so, we also acquire great ideals for life. These may not extend to cosmic dimensions but instead, basically, relate to the question of why we come together in an anthroposophical society. To understand the purpose of this society, we need to return once more to the idea that we work for the Spirits of Personality, for the Time Spirit. When we enter this world at birth we are first brought up and educated by the most diverse circumstances. These work upon us, forming the prelude to our own self-creative activity. It would be so helpful for people to realize that the fact they are born in a particular place, and that particular circumstances work upon them, is indeed a prelude, a preparatory stage. These circumstances exert a suggestive influence. Let us try to imagine how differently a person would be affected by being born, say, in Rome or Frankfurt instead of Constantinople. His circumstances would be different, also as regards religion, which accordingly might lead him to become a somewhat fanatical Catholic or Protestant. But if a small cog had turned in the karmic continuum and he was born in Constantinople instead, he might well become a proper Turk. Here's just one example of the suggestive way in which environmental circumstances can work on us. But we can work our way out of merely suggestive conditions and unite with others in accord with self-chosen insights and principles, knowing *why* we are working with these other people. Then, from our conscious awareness arise social connections in which material is created for the Spirits of Time, of Personality. The Anthroposophical Society is one such, a context of interrelationships founded on fraternity. This means nothing other than each person working to create the society by acquiring, on a small scale, all the good qualities which make him a reflection of the society as a whole. In other words, he offers up the ideas, the richness of feelings and virtues he develops through the society as sustenance to the Spirits of Personality.

A society of this kind combines what creates human coexistence with the principle of individuality. Through such a society each individual is rendered capable of offering up to the Spirits of Personality what he produces or creates. And each member works towards the perspective adopted by its most advanced proponents, whose spiritual schooling has led them to embrace the following ideal: 'When I think I do not do so for my own satisfaction, but so that the Spirits of Personality may draw sustenance from my thoughts. I place my best, my most beautiful thoughts upon the altar of the Spirits of Personality. And what I feel is not felt out of egoism but rather I feel so that this may be nourishment for the Spirits of Personality. And likewise, the virtues I manage to practise I do not practise in order to be highly regarded but to offer up my sacrifice, to create sustenance for the Spirits of Personality.' In seeking to do this we make our ideal those we call the Masters of Wisdom and of the Harmony of Feelings. For this is the way they think, preparing a form of human evolution which will increasingly enable us to create ever new things, and ultimately to evolve a world of effects from which all old causes have vanished, and from which a new light shines out towards the future. The world is not subject to continuous change in which it assumes entirely different forms but instead the old perfects itself, and this improvement to the old becomes the vehicle of the new. Then, however, this vehicle is cast away and vanishes into nothing so that the new can emerge from this nothing. This is the mighty idea of progress, in which something new can always and continually arise.

But worlds are self-contained, and you have seen from the example I have given that we cannot in fact speak of the ultimate demise of anything. We have seen how the Spirits of Personality lose their effect on us, on the one hand, but on the other take up their evolution again; and so we have a world that always rejuvenates itself, but of which we can say that whatever is cast off would prevent further progress and instead is bestowed upon another so that he in turn can progress. No one should believe he must inevitably let something fall away into nothing because he has been endowed with the capacity to create out of nothing. But what will appear as the new on Vulcan will continually create new forms and cast off the old; and what is cast off in this way will seek its own further path.

Unfolding, infolding and creation from nothing are the three concepts by means of which we should seek to understand the true nature of the development of the world and its phenomena. Only by this means do we properly arrive at concepts that explain the world to us and give us feelings of inwardness. You see, if a person has to tell himself that he can only create what is implanted in him as cause, and this alone can come to expression in him, this idea will be unable to steel his powers and kindle his hope to the same extent as realizing he can create living values, and continually add new elements to the foundations given to him. We can then see that the old will not prevent us from creating new blossoms and fruits that survive into the future. And this is a part of what we can characterize by saying that the anthroposophical world view gives people living forces, living hope and confidence for life by showing them that they can help shape the future not only of things arising from the realm of causation but of others that as yet do not exist, that lie in the realm of nothing; and this, truly, offers us the prospect of working our way from being a creature to being a creator.

NOTES

Original sources: These lectures were given in the winter half year 1908/1909 at the Besant branch of the Theosophical Society in Berlin. They formed part, and were a continuation of, ongoing studies which at that time had lasted over seven years in this group.

Original texts: The lectures were recorded in shorthand by several members of the audience, of whom we only know Walter Vegelahn and Franz Seiler by name, and then written up in full. The published version is based on these texts. Only Franz Seiler's original shorthand versions still exist and some of these are deficient in places. For the third (German) edition (1973) the text was revised with the aid of new, more detailed transcripts which had since found their way into the archive of Rudolf Steiner's literary estate.

The lecture titles are likely to be by Rudolf Steiner. Some were announced beforehand in the 'Newsletter for members of the German section of the Theosophical Society' (ed. Mathilde Scholl).

The volume title of the original German: It is not known who formulated this, but it is very likely to have been approved by Rudolf Steiner when the first edition was published in 1915.

When Rudolf Steiner gave these lectures, his anthroposophically oriented spiritual science was still integrated into the Theosophical Society of that time. Steiner used the terms 'theosophy' and 'theosophical', but from the beginning did so with an anthroposophical orientation. In line with a later suggestion by Steiner, these terms have been replaced by 'spiritual science' or 'anthroposophy'.

Titles of works not available in their entirety in English are given in the original German.

1. Annual general meeting on 26 October 1908.
2. The two first lecture series in the Theosophical Library in Berlin took place during the winter of 1900/01 and 1901/02 under the respective titles of 'Mysticism' and 'Christianity as Mystical Fact'. These subsequently gave rise to two books by Rudolf Steiner: *Eleven European Mystics*, RSP, 1971, GA 7; and *Christianity as Mystical Fact and the Mysteries of Antiquity*, SteinerBooks, 2006, GA 8.
3. See the Berlin lectures from January 1908 onwards, published in the volume *Das Hereinwirken geistiger Wesenheiten in den Menschen*, GA 102 (not available in entirety in English).
4. Friedrich Nietzsche (1844–1900) suffered a breakdown in early January 1889 in Turin.
5. The meaning but not a literal rendering of Nietzsche's letter to Jacob Burckhardt, dated 6 January 1889.

6. Again, the meaning but not a literal rendering of a passage in Friedrich Nietzsche's *Ecce homo*, 'The Twilight of the Idols', § 3.

7. In the letter referred to above to Jacob Burckhardt.

8. Quote from Goethe's poem, 'Vermächtnis' ('Bequest').

9. The annual general meeting itself did not take place for another week, on 26 October 1908, but various events were always held leading up to and around the time of the general meeting.

10. In 'Goethe's Scientific Writings', edited with commentaries by Rudolf Steiner in Kuerschner's *Deutsche National-Litteratur* (1884/97), 5 vols, reprinted Dornach 1975, GA 1a–e, vol. I: *Bildung und Umbildung organischer Naturen, Die Metamorphose der Pflanzen*, pp. 17ff.

11. Lecture of 22 October 1908 on the fourth dimension, published in GA 324a, *The Fourth Dimension—Sacred Geometry, Alchemy and Mathematics* (Anthroposophic Press, 2001).

12. See lectures in the volumes *Das christliche Mysterium*, GA 97, *Menschheitsentwicklung und Christus-Erkenntnis*, GA 100, and *The Gospel of St John*, GA 103, Anthroposophic Press, 1940.

13. Homer, *The Odyssey*, XI, canto 489–491.

14. Translator's note: This series of articles first appeared in the journal *Lucifer-Gnosis* between 1904 and 1908, and was published in 1909 as GA 10 (*Knowledge of the Higher Worlds*).

15. Two public lectures in the Architektenhaus: on 22 October 1908 on 'Goethe's Secret Revelation (exoteric)', and on 24 October 1908 on 'Goethe's Secret Revelation (esoteric)'. These were published in GA 57, *Wo und wie findet man den Geist?* They were published in English as *Goethe's Secret Revelation*, Percy, Lund, Humphries & Co, 1933. See also Rudolf Steiner's essay 'Goethes geheime Offenbarung. Zu seinem hundertfünfzigsten Geburtstage: 28. August 1899', published in *Methodische Grundlagen der Anthroposophie. Gesammelte Aufsätze 1884–1901*, GA 30; and the later book *Goethes Geistesart in ihrer Offenbarung durch seinen 'Faust' und durch das Märchen von der Schlange und der Lilie*, GA 22.

16. Savonarola, 1452–98: a Dominican, reformer of the order and, under the auspices of the Borgia Pope Alexander IV, a successful preacher on morals and repentance in Florence. On the same day that Rudolf Steiner gave this lecture, he also gave another members' lecture on 'The Mission of Savonarola', published in GA 108.

17. Rudolf Steiner had often spoken of the human group souls, in particular in connection with the seals of the Apocalypse of St John. Cf. GA 284/285, *Rosicrucianism Renewed—The Unity of Art, Science & Religion: The Theosophical Congress of Whitsun 1907*, SteinerBooks 2007; and GA 104, *The Apocalypse of St John*, RSP, 1985.

18. For instance, in a 1909 work on 'inheritance and memory' by Gustav Eichhorn, a copy of which was in Rudolf Steiner's library; and a 1908 book on the 'soul life of plants' by Gustav Theodor, which Steiner mentions elsewhere.

19. *Faust*, Part I: 'Study'. Verse 1740. See the lecture of the same title given in Berlin on 25 October 1906, published in *Supersensible Knowledge*, GA 55, Anthroposophic Press, 1987.

20. Paracelsus, 1493–1541. Theophrastus Bombastus Paracelsus of Hohenheim. A great doctor, philosopher and researcher of the natural world, he was born at Einsiedeln, Schwyz (Switzerland), and embarked on wide-ranging travels and studies. Trithem of Sponheim is thought to have been one of his teachers. Between 1526 and 1528 he was city physician in Basel and professor at the university, but had to leave the city due to disputes with the municipal authorities and other physicians. From then on he lived an erratic life in various locations in southern Germany, often in great poverty, but during this period wrote his great medical and chemical texts before dying in Salzburg. Rudolf Steiner gave detailed attention to Paracelsus and repeatedly spoke of his life and work in books, public lectures and members' lectures. Cf. in particular the chapter 'Agrippa of Nettesheim and Theophrastus Paracelsus' in Rudolf Steiner, *Eleven European Mystics* (GA 7) RSP, 1971, and 'Paracelsus', a public lecture given in Berlin on 26 April 1906, published in *Die Welträtsel und die Anthroposophie*, GA 54; and 'Von Paracelsus zu Goethe', public lecture given in Berlin on 9 November 1911, published in *Menschengeschichte im Lichte der Geistesforschung*, GA 61. See also: Johannes Hemleben, *Paracelsus. Revolutionär, Arzt und Christ*, Stuttgart 1972.
21. Paracelsus, *Opus paramirum*, Book 3, Tract 2.
22. Berlin, 12 and 14 November 1908, published in *Wo und wie findet man den Geist?* GA 57.
23. See the lecture 'The Bible and Wisdom I', Berlin, 12 November 1908, op. cit.
24. Genesis 2:4 in Rudolf Steiner's translation. Cf. the lecture cited above, 'The Bible and Wisdom I'.
25. Genesis 5:1.
26. Exodus 3:14.
27. Cf. Exodus 3:6.
28. Exodus 3:14.
29. Exodus 23, 25–6.
30. Rudolf Steiner is probably referring to a pamphlet in his library by Dr Ludwig Wulff-Parchim, entitled *Dekalog und Vaterunser* ('The Ten Commandments and the Lord's Prayer'), Parchim 1907. The passage he quotes is however not found in that volume in quite that form.
31. The lecture of 10 November 1908, the eighth in this volume.
32. Lecture of 16 November 1908, the ninth lecture in this volume.
33. Arthur Schopenhauer, 1788–1860. In relation to this statement cf. *The World as Will and Idea*, Book 4, § 55.
34. The 18 public lectures given in the Architektenhaus in Berlin, from 15 October 1908 to 6 May 1909, published as *Wo und wie finde ich den Geist?* GA 57.
35. Berlin, 10 December 1908, in GA 57.
36. Rudolf Steiner spoke on this theme in various places in 1906, initially in Berlin on 16 April of that year at the time Vesuvius erupted. See GA 96: *Original Impulses for the Science of the Spirit*, Completion Press, 2001.
37. Rudolf Steiner spoke on very numerous occasions about Goethe and his *Faust*. He spoke at length about the scenes with the Mothers in GA 272 and 273, which are not at present available in English.

38. *Faust* Part II, Act One, Dark Gallery, verse 6275.
39. *Faust* Part II, Act One, Dark Gallery, verse 6256.
40. Lecture of 28 December 1908, of which only brief notes survive—which show that Steiner was speaking here of the Atlantean mysteries.
41. *Faust* Part I, Auerbach's Cellar in Leipzig, verse 2181.
42. See lecture of 22 March 1909 in this volume, pp. 194f.
43. See note 36 above.
44. Refers to the lecture of 21 December 1908, the eleventh in this volume.
45. See note 44 above.
46. See note 34 above.
47. Refers to lecture 8 in this volume.
48. Matthew 18:3.
49. Lecture of 28 December 1908. No transcript of this exists, since transcribing was not permitted for this lecture. A few points later written down from memory by someone present shows that the theme was the same as one subsequently explored elsewhere and published in GA 109/111, *Das Prinzip der spirituellen Ökonomie*.
50. Genesis 6.
51. Irenaeus, Bishop of Lyon in 177/78. In Smyrna, as a boy, he had heard the sermons of the bishop and martyr Polycarp who, like Papias, was thought to have been a pupil of the Apostles. See Fragment 12 in J.P. Migne, *Patrologia Graeca*, vol. 7, p. 1227. In his work attacking the Gnostics, *Adversus haereses*, Irenaeus describes the unbroken succession of apostles and bishops (apostolic succession) as a guarantee of the truth of Christian doctrine.
52. Born AD 70, Papias was Bishop of Hierapolis in Phrygia and had probably been a pupil of the Apostle John and a companion of Polycarp.
53. Augustine of Hippo, 354–430. The citation is freely rendered from Contr. epist. Manich 5. The original runs: 'Evangelio non crederem, nisi me ecclesiae commoveret auctoritas.' Quoted in Otto Wilimann, *Geschichte des Idealismus*, vol. II, Braunschweig 1896, p. 256.
54. Old Saxon Biblical paraphrase poem, in alliterative verse, composed between AD 822 and 840. The author is unknown but was probably a cleric from the Fuldar School. See also Rudolf Steiner's comments in his lecture of 26 March 1924 in Dornach, in GA 353: *From Beetroot to Buddhism, 16 discussions with workers*, RSP, 1999.
55. Francis of Assisi, 1182–1226.
56. Elisabeth of Thuringia, 1207–31.
57. Meister Eckhart, 1260–1327; Johannes Tauler, 1300–61.
58. Matthew 26:26 and 28.
59. Nicolaus Copernicus, 1473–1543; Giordano Bruno, 1548–1600.
60. Ernst Haeckel, 1834–1919; Charles Darwin, 1809–82; Emil Du Bois-Reymond, 1815–96; Thomas Henry Huxley, 1825–95; David Friedrich Strauss, 1808–74.
61. 'Be not deceived; God is not mocked: for whatsoever a man soweth, that shall he also reap.' Galatians, 6:7.
62. This treatise on education appeared in 1907 in issue 33 of the journal *Lucifer-Gnosis* that Steiner edited. This is republished in the collected works as GA 34.

63. Genesis 3:16.
64. Exodus 3:14.
65. See note 13 above.
66. See, for instance, Mark 13:11 and John 14:26.
67. These are beings of great significance for humanity's evolution: 'These lofty beings have already accomplished the path which the rest of humanity must still take. They now work as the great teachers of wisdom and of the harmony of humanity's feelings.' (From a letter by Rudolf Steiner to a member, Berlin, 20 January 1905, published in GA 264: *From the History and Contents of the First Section of the Esoteric School 1904–1914*). See also the commentary by the editor of GA 264, Hella Wiesberger, in the appendix to that volume, on 'The Masters of Wisdom and of the Harmony of Feelings in the work of Rudolf Steiner'.
68. The passage, literally translated, is: 'For were I a king and knew it not myself, then were I no king.' In: Meister Eckhart, *Deutsche Predigten und Traktate*, edited and translated from Latin by Josef Quint, Munich 1963, Zurich 1979. Sermon 36: 'Sciote, quia prope est regnum dei (Luc 21, 31)'.
69. See also Chapter II of GA 264, *From the History and Contents of the First Section of the Esoteric School 1904–1914*: 'The History of the division of the Esoteric School of Theosophy into an eastern and a western school in 1907'.
70. Rudolf Steiner is here referring to H.P. Blavatsky, *The Secret Doctrine*, vol. 3, footnote to p. 89 in the German edition.
71. This passage relates to H.P. Blavatsky's dismissal of this esoteric fact in her book *The Secret Doctrine*, vol. 3.
72. Rudolf Steiner is here again referring to H.P. Blavatsky's *The Secret Doctrine*, vol. 3, section XLIII, 'The Mystery of the Buddha'. Shankaracharya, AD 788–820 was a reformer of the Vedas and of other Indian wisdom.
73. See lecture given in Berlin on 23 January 1908, 'The Soul of the Animals in the Light of Spiritual Science': lecture 8 in GA 56, *Die Erkenntnis der Seele und des Geistes*.
74. Lecture in Berlin on 4 March 1909 in GA 56 (see note above). Cf. also 'The Mystery of the Human Temperaments', Basel 1975.
75. Genesis 2:7. Translator's note: In the King James version, this is called 'the breath of life'.
76. The Iliad, canto 6, verse 484.

RUDOLF STEINER'S COLLECTED WORKS

The German Edition of Rudolf Steiner's Collected Works (the *Gesamtausgabe* [GA] published by Rudolf Steiner Verlag, Dornach, Switzerland) presently runs to 354 titles, organized either by type of work (written or spoken), chronology, audience (public or other), or subject (education, art, etc.). For ease of comparison, the Collected Works in English [CW] follows the German organization exactly. A complete listing of the CWs follows with literal translations of the German titles. Other than in the case of the books published in his lifetime, titles were rarely given by Rudolf Steiner himself, and were often provided by the editors of the German editions. The titles in English are not necessarily the same as the German; and, indeed, over the past seventy-five years have frequently been different, with the same book sometimes appearing under different titles.

For ease of identification and to avoid confusion, we suggest that readers looking for a title should do so by CW number. Because the work of creating the Collected Works of Rudolf Steiner is an ongoing process, with new titles being published every year, we have not indicated in this listing which books are presently available. To find out what titles in the Collected Works are currently in print, please check our website at www.rudolfsteinerpress.com (or www.steinerbooks.org for US readers).

Written Work

CW 1	Goethe: Natural-Scientific Writings, Introduction, with Footnotes and Explanations in the text by Rudolf Steiner
CW 2	Outlines of an Epistemology of the Goethean World View, with Special Consideration of Schiller
CW 3	Truth and Science
CW 4	The Philosophy of Freedom
CW 4a	Documents to 'The Philosophy of Freedom'
CW 5	Friedrich Nietzsche, A Fighter against His Own Time
CW 6	Goethe's Worldview
CW 6a	Now in CW 30
CW 7	Mysticism at the Dawn of Modern Spiritual Life and Its Relationship with Modern Worldviews
CW 8	Christianity as Mystical Fact and the Mysteries of Antiquity
CW 9	Theosophy: An Introduction into Supersensible World Knowledge and Human Purpose
CW 10	How Does One Attain Knowledge of Higher Worlds?
CW 11	From the Akasha-Chronicle

CW 12   Levels of Higher Knowledge

CW 13   Occult Science in Outline

CW 14   Four Mystery Dramas

CW 15   The Spiritual Guidance of the Individual and Humanity

CW 16   A Way to Human Self-Knowledge: Eight Meditations

CW 17   The Threshold of the Spiritual World. Aphoristic Comments

CW 18   The Riddles of Philosophy in Their History, Presented as an Outline

CW 19   Contained in CW 24

CW 20   The Riddles of the Human Being: Articulated and Unarticulated in the Thinking, Views and Opinions of a Series of German and Austrian Personalities

CW 21   The Riddles of the Soul

CW 22   Goethe's Spiritual Nature And Its Revelation In 'Faust' and through the 'Fairy Tale of the Snake and the Lily'

CW 23   The Central Points of the Social Question in the Necessities of Life in the Present and the Future

CW 24   Essays Concerning the Threefold Division of the Social Organism and the Period 1915–1921

CW 25   Cosmology, Religion and Philosophy

CW 26   Anthroposophical Leading Thoughts

CW 27   Fundamentals for Expansion of the Art of Healing according to Spiritual-Scientific Insights

CW 28   The Course of My Life

CW 29   Collected Essays on Dramaturgy, 1889–1900

CW 30   Methodical Foundations of Anthroposophy: Collected Essays on Philosophy, Natural Science, Aesthetics and Psychology, 1884–1901

CW 31   Collected Essays on Culture and Current Events, 1887–1901

CW 32   Collected Essays on Literature, 1884–1902

CW 33   Biographies and Biographical Sketches, 1894–1905

CW 34   Lucifer-Gnosis: Foundational Essays on Anthroposophy and Reports from the Periodicals 'Lucifer' and 'Lucifer-Gnosis,' 1903–1908

CW 35   Philosophy and Anthroposophy: Collected Essays, 1904–1923

CW 36   The Goetheanum-Idea in the Middle of the Cultural Crisis of the Present: Collected Essays from the Periodical 'Das Goetheanum,' 1921–1925

CW 37   Now in CWs 260a and 251

CW 38   Letters, Vol. 1: 1881–1890

CW 39   Letters, Vol. 2: 1890–1925

CW 40   Truth-Wrought Words

CW 40a   Sayings, Poems and Mantras; Supplementary Volume

CW 42   Now in CWs 264–266

CW 43   Stage Adaptations

CW 44   On the Four Mystery Dramas. Sketches, Fragments and Paralipomena on the Four Mystery Dramas

CW 45   Anthroposophy: A Fragment from the Year 1910

Public Lectures

CW 51	On Philosophy, History and Literature
CW 52	Spiritual Teachings Concerning the Soul and Observation of the World
CW 53	The Origin and Goal of the Human Being
CW 54	The Riddles of the World and Anthroposophy
CW 55	Knowledge of the Supersensible in Our Times and Its Meaning for Life Today
CW 56	Knowledge of the Soul and of the Spirit
CW 57	Where and How Does One Find the Spirit?
CW 58	The Metamorphoses of the Soul Life. Paths of Soul Experiences: Part One
CW 59	The Metamorphoses of the Soul Life. Paths of Soul Experiences: Part Two
CW 60	The Answers of Spiritual Science to the Biggest Questions of Existence
CW 61	Human History in the Light of Spiritual Research
CW 62	Results of Spiritual Research
CW 63	Spiritual Science as a Treasure for Life
CW 64	Out of Destiny-Burdened Times
CW 65	Out of Central European Spiritual Life
CW 66	Spirit and Matter, Life and Death
CW 67	The Eternal in the Human Soul. Immortality and Freedom
CW 68	Public lectures in various cities, 1906–1918
CW 69	Public lectures in various cities, 1906–1918
CW 70	Public lectures in various cities, 1906–1918
CW 71	Public lectures in various cities, 1906–1918
CW 72	Freedom—Immortality—Social Life
CW 73	The Supplementing of the Modern Sciences through Anthroposophy
CW 73a	Specialized Fields of Knowledge and Anthroposophy
CW 74	The Philosophy of Thomas Aquinas
CW 75	Public lectures in various cities, 1906–1918
CW 76	The Fructifying Effect of Anthroposophy on Specialized Fields
CW 77a	The Task of Anthroposophy in Relation to Science and Life: The Darmstadt College Course
CW 77b	Art and Anthroposophy. The Goetheanum-Impulse
CW 78	Anthroposophy, Its Roots of Knowledge and Fruits for Life
CW 79	The Reality of the Higher Worlds
CW 80	Public lectures in various cities, 1922
CW 81	Renewal-Impulses for Culture and Science—Berlin College Course
CW 82	So that the Human Being Can Become a Complete Human Being
CW 83	Western and Eastern World-Contrast. Paths to Understanding It through Anthroposophy
CW 84	What Did the Goetheanum Intend and What Should Anthroposophy Do?

Lectures to the Members of the Anthroposophical Society

CW 88   Concerning the Astral World and Devachan

CW 89   Consciousness—Life—Form. Fundamental Principles of a Spiritual-Scientific Cosmology

CW 90   Participant Notes from the Lectures during the Years 1903–1905

CW 91   Participant Notes from the Lectures during the Years 1903–1905

CW 92   The Occult Truths of Ancient Myths and Sagas

CW 93   The Temple Legend and the Golden Legend

CW 93a   Fundamentals of Esotericism

CW 94   Cosmogony. Popular Occultism. The Gospel of John. The Theosophy in the Gospel of John

CW 95   At the Gates of Theosophy

CW 96   Origin-Impulses of Spiritual Science. Christian Esotericism in the Light of New Spirit-Knowledge

CW 97   The Christian Mystery

CW 98   Nature Beings and Spirit Beings—Their Effects in Our Visible World

CW 99   The Theosophy of the Rosicrucians

CW 100   Human Development and Christ-Knowledge

CW 101   Myths and Legends. Occult Signs and Symbols

CW 102   The Working into Human Beings by Spiritual Beings

CW 103   The Gospel of John

CW 104   The Apocalypse of John

CW 104a   From the Picture-Script of the Apocalypse of John

CW 105   Universe, Earth, the Human Being: Their Being and Development, as well as Their Reflection in the Connection between Egyptian Mythology and Modern Culture

CW 106   Egyptian Myths and Mysteries in Relation to the Active Spiritual Forces of the Present

CW 107   Spiritual-Scientific Knowledge of the Human Being

CW 108   Answering the Questions of Life and the World through Anthroposophy

CW 109   The Principle of Spiritual Economy in Connection with the Question of Reincarnation. An Aspect of the Spiritual Guidance of Humanity

CW 110   The Spiritual Hierarchies and Their Reflection in the Physical World. Zodiac, Planets and Cosmos

CW 111   Contained in CW 109

CW 112   The Gospel of John in Relation to the Three Other Gospels, Especially the Gospel of Luke

CW 113   The Orient in the Light of the Occident. The Children of Lucifer and the Brothers of Christ

CW 114   The Gospel of Luke

CW 115   Anthroposophy—Psychosophy—Pneumatosophy

CW 116   The Christ-Impulse and the Development of 'I'-Consciousness

CW 117   The Deeper Secrets of the Development of Humanity in Light of the Gospels

CW 118   The Event of the Christ-Appearance in the Etheric World

CW 119   Macrocosm and Microcosm. The Large World and the Small World. Soul-Questions, Life-Questions, Spirit-Questions

CW 120   The Revelation of Karma

CW 121   The Mission of Individual Folk-Souls in Connection with Germanic-Nordic Mythology

CW 122   The Secrets of the Biblical Creation-Story. The Six-Day Work in the First Book of Moses

CW 123   The Gospel of Matthew

CW 124   Excursus in the Area of the Gospel of Mark

CW 125   Paths and Goals of the Spiritual Human Being. Life Questions in the Light of Spiritual Science

CW 126   Occult History. Esoteric Observations of the Karmic Relationships of Personalities and Events of World History

CW 127   The Mission of the New Spiritual Revelation. The Christ-Event as the Middle-Point of Earth Evolution

CW 128   An Occult Physiology

CW 129   Wonders of the World, Trials of the Soul, and Revelations of the Spirit

CW 130   Esoteric Christianity and the Spiritual Guidance of Humanity

CW 131   From Jesus to Christ

CW 132   Evolution from the View Point of the Truth

CW 133   The Earthly and the Cosmic Human Being

CW 134   The World of the Senses and the World of the Spirit

CW 135   Reincarnation and Karma and their Meaning for the Culture of the Present

CW 136   The Spiritual Beings in Celestial Bodies and the Realms of Nature

CW 137   The Human Being in the Light of Occultism, Theosophy and Philosophy

CW 138   On Initiation. On Eternity and the Passing Moment. On the Light of the Spirit and the Darkness of Life

CW 139   The Gospel of Mark

CW 140   Occult Investigation into the Life between Death and New Birth. The Living Interaction between Life and Death

CW 141   Life between Death and New Birth in Relationship to Cosmic Facts

CW 142   The Bhagavad Gita and the Letters of Paul

CW 143   Experiences of the Supersensible. Three Paths of the Soul to Christ

CW 144   The Mysteries of the East and of Christianity

CW 145   What Significance Does Occult Development of the Human Being Have for the Sheaths—Physical Body, Etheric Body, Astral Body, and Self?

CW 146   The Occult Foundations of the Bhagavad Gita

CW 147   The Secrets of the Threshold

CW 148   Out of Research in the Akasha: The Fifth Gospel

CW 149   Christ and the Spiritual World. Concerning the Search for the Holy Grail

CW 150	The World of the Spirit and Its Extension into Physical Existence; The Influence of the Dead in the World of the Living
CW 151	Human Thought and Cosmic Thought
CW 152	Preliminary Stages to the Mystery of Golgotha
CW 153	The Inner Being of the Human Being and Life Between Death and New Birth
CW 154	How does One Gain an Understanding of the Spiritual World? The Flowing in of Spiritual Impulses from out of the World of the Deceased
CW 155	Christ and the Human Soul. Concerning the Meaning of Life. Theosophical Morality. Anthroposophy and Christianity
CW 156	Occult Reading and Occult Hearing
CW 157	Human Destinies and the Destiny of Peoples
CW 157a	The Formation of Destiny and the Life after Death
CW 158	The Connection Between the Human Being and the Elemental World. Kalevala—Olaf Asteson—The Russian People—The World as the Result of the Influences of Equilibrium
CW 159	The Mystery of Death. The Nature and Significance of Middle Europe and the European Folk Spirits
CW 160	In CW 159
CW 161	Paths of Spiritual Knowledge and the Renewal of the Artistic Worldview
CW 162	Questions of Art and Life in Light of Spiritual Science
CW 163	Coincidence, Necessity and Providence. Imaginative Knowledge and the Processes after Death
CW 164	The Value of Thinking for a Knowledge That Satisfies the Human Being. The Relationship of Spiritual Science to Natural Science
CW 165	The Spiritual Unification of Humanity through the Christ-Impulse
CW 166	Necessity and Freedom in the Events of the World and in Human Action
CW 167	The Present and the Past in the Human Spirit
CW 168	The Connection between the Living and the Dead
CW 169	World-being and Selfhood
CW 170	The Riddle of the Human Being. The Spiritual Background of Human History. Cosmic and Human History, Vol. 1
CW 171	Inner Development-Impulses of Humanity. Goethe and the Crisis of the 19th Century. Cosmic and Human History, Vol. 2
CW 172	The Karma of the Vocation of the Human Being in Connection with Goethe's Life. Cosmic and Human History, Vol. 3
CW 173	Contemporary-Historical Considerations: The Karma of Untruthfulness, Part One. Cosmic and Human History, Vol. 4
CW 174	Contemporary-Historical Considerations: The Karma of Untruthfulness, Part Two. Cosmic and Human History, Vol. 5
CW 174a	Middle Europe between East and West. Cosmic and Human History, Vol. 6
CW 174b	The Spiritual Background of the First World War. Cosmic and Human History, Vol. 7

CW 175   Building Stones for an Understanding of the Mystery of Golgotha. Cosmic and Human Metamorphoses

CW 176   Truths of Evolution of the Individual and Humanity. The Karma of Materialism

CW 177   The Spiritual Background of the Outer World. The Fall of the Spirits of Darkness. Spiritual Beings and Their Effects, Vol. 1

CW 178   Individual Spiritual Beings and their Influence in the Soul of the Human Being. Spiritual Beings and their Effects, Vol. 2

CW 179   Spiritual Beings and Their Effects. Historical Necessity and Freedom. The Influences on Destiny from out of the World of the Dead. Spiritual Beings and Their Effects, Vol. 3

CW 180   Mystery Truths and Christmas Impulses. Ancient Myths and their Meaning. Spiritual Beings and Their Effects, Vol. 4

CW 181   Earthly Death and Cosmic Life. Anthroposophical Gifts for Life. Necessities of Consciousness for the Present and the Future.

CW 182   Death as Transformation of Life

CW 183   The Science of the Development of the Human Being

CW 184   The Polarity of Duration and Development in Human Life. The Cosmic Pre-History of Humanity

CW 185   Historical Symptomology

CW 185a   Historical-Developmental Foundations for Forming a Social Judgment

CW 186   The Fundamental Social Demands of Our Time—In Changed Situations

CW 187   How Can Humanity Find the Christ Again? The Threefold Shadow-Existence of our Time and the New Christ-Light

CW 188   Goetheanism, a Transformation-Impulse and Resurrection-Thought. Science of the Human Being and Science of Sociology

CW 189   The Social Question as a Question of Consciousness. The Spiritual Background of the Social Question, Vol. 1

CW 190   Impulses of the Past and the Future in Social Occurrences. The Spiritual Background of the Social Question, Vol. 2

CW 191   Social Understanding from Spiritual-Scientific Cognition. The Spiritual Background of the Social Question, Vol. 3

CW 192   Spiritual-Scientific Treatment of Social and Pedagogical Questions

CW 193   The Inner Aspect of the Social Riddle. Luciferic Past and Ahrimanic Future

CW 194   The Mission of Michael. The Revelation of the Actual Mysteries of the Human Being

CW 195   Cosmic New Year and the New Year Idea

CW 196   Spiritual and Social Transformations in the Development of Humanity

CW 197   Polarities in the Development of Humanity: West and East Materialism and Mysticism Knowledge and Belief

CW 198   Healing Factors for the Social Organism

CW 199   Spiritual Science as Knowledge of the Foundational Impulses of Social Formation

CW 200   The New Spirituality and the Christ-Experience of the 20th Century

CW 201   The Correspondences Between Microcosm and Macrocosm. The Human Being—A Hieroglyph of the Universe. The Human Being in Relationship with the Cosmos: 1

CW 202   The Bridge between the World-Spirituality and the Physical Aspect of the Human Being. The Search for the New Isis, the Divine Sophia. The Human Being in Relationship with the Cosmos: 2

CW 203   The Responsibility of Human Beings for the Development of the World through their Spiritual Connection with the Planet Earth and the World of the Stars. The Human Being in Relationship with the Cosmos: 3

CW 204   Perspectives of the Development of Humanity. The Materialistic Knowledge-Impulse and the Task of Anthroposophy. The Human Being in Relationship with the Cosmos: 4

CW 205   Human Development, World-Soul, and World-Spirit. Part One: The Human Being as a Being of Body and Soul in Relationship to the World. The Human Being in Relationship with the Cosmos: 5

CW 206   Human Development, World-Soul, and World-Spirit. Part Two: The Human Being as a Spiritual Being in the Process of Historical Development. The Human Being in Relationship with the Cosmos: 6

CW 207   Anthroposophy as Cosmosophy. Part One: Characteristic Features of the Human Being in the Earthly and the Cosmic Realms. The Human Being in Relationship with the Cosmos: 7

CW 208   Anthroposophy as Cosmosophy. Part Two: The Forming of the Human Being as the Result of Cosmic Influence. The Human Being in Relationship with the Cosmos: 8

CW 209   Nordic and Central European Spiritual Impulses. The Festival of the Appearance of Christ. The Human Being in Relationship with the Cosmos: 9

CW 210   Old and New Methods of Initiation. Drama and Poetry in the Change of Consciousness in the Modern Age

CW 211   The Sun Mystery and the Mystery of Death and Resurrection. Exoteric and Esoteric Christianity

CW 212   Human Soul Life and Spiritual Striving in Connection with World and Earth Development

CW 213   Human Questions and World Answers

CW 214   The Mystery of the Trinity: The Human Being in Relationship with the Spiritual World in the Course of Time

CW 215   Philosophy, Cosmology, and Religion in Anthroposophy

CW 216   The Fundamental Impulses of the World-Historical Development of Humanity

CW 217   Spiritually Active Forces in the Coexistence of the Older and Younger Generations. Pedagogical Course for Youth

CW 217a   Youth's Cognitive Task

CW 218   Spiritual Connections in the Forming of the Human Organism

CW 219   The Relationship of the World of the Stars to the Human Being, and of the Human Being to the World of the Stars. The Spiritual Communion of Humanity

CW 220   Living Knowledge of Nature. Intellectual Fall and Spiritual Redemption

CW 221   Earth-Knowing and Heaven-Insight

CW 222   The Imparting of Impulses to World-Historical Events through Spiritual Powers

CW 223   The Cycle of the Year as Breathing Process of the Earth and the Four Great Festival-Seasons. Anthroposophy and the Human Heart (Gemüt)

CW 224   The Human Soul and its Connection with Divine-Spiritual Individualities. The Internalization of the Festivals of the Year

CW 225   Three Perspectives of Anthroposophy. Cultural Phenomena observed from a Spiritual-Scientific Perspective

CW 226   Human Being, Human Destiny, and World Development

CW 227   Initiation-Knowledge

CW 228   Science of Initiation and Knowledge of the Stars. The Human Being in the Past, the Present, and the Future from the Viewpoint of the Development of Consciousness

CW 229   The Experiencing of the Course of the Year in Four Cosmic Imaginations

CW 230   The Human Being as Harmony of the Creative, Building, and Formative World-Word

CW 231   The Supersensible Human Being, Understood Anthroposophically

CW 232   The Forming of the Mysteries

CW 233   World History Illuminated by Anthroposophy and as the Foundation for Knowledge of the Human Spirit

CW 233a   Mystery Sites of the Middle Ages: Rosicrucianism and the Modern Initiation-Principle. The Festival of Easter as Part of the History of the Mysteries of Humanity

CW 234   Anthroposophy. A Summary after 21 Years

CW 235   Esoteric Observations of Karmic Relationships in 6 Volumes, Vol. 1

CW 236   Esoteric Observations of Karmic Relationships in 6 Volumes, Vol. 2

CW 237   Esoteric Observations of Karmic Relationships in 6 Volumes, Vol. 3:
The Karmic Relationships of the Anthroposophical Movement

CW 238   Esoteric Observations of Karmic Relationships in 6 Volumes, Vol. 4:
The Spiritual Life of the Present in Relationship to the Anthroposophical Movement

CW 239   Esoteric Observations of Karmic Relationships in 6 Volumes, Vol. 5

CW 240   Esoteric Observations of Karmic Relationships in 6 Volumes, Vol. 6

CW 243   The Consciousness of the Initiate

CW 245   Instructions for an Esoteric Schooling

CW 250   The Building-Up of the Anthroposophical Society. From the Beginning to the Outbreak of the First World War

CW 251   The History of the Goetheanum Building-Association

CW 252   Life in the Anthroposophical Society from the First World War to the Burning of the First Goetheanum

CW 253   The Problems of Living Together in the Anthroposophical Society. On the Dornach Crisis of 1915. With Highlights on Swedenborg's Clairvoyance, the Views of Freudian Psychoanalysts, and the Concept of Love in Relation to Mysticism

CW 254   The Occult Movement in the 19th Century and Its Relationship to World Culture. Significant Points from the Exoteric Cultural Life around the Middle of the 19th Century

CW 255   Rudolf Steiner during the First World War

CW 255a   Anthroposophy and the Reformation of Society. On the History of the Threefold Movement

CW 255b   Anthroposophy and Its Opponents, 1919–1921

CW 256   How Can the Anthroposophical Movement Be Financed?

CW 256a   Futurum, Inc. / International Laboratories, Inc.

CW 256b   The Coming Day, Inc.

CW 257   Anthroposophical Community-Building

CW 258   The History of and Conditions for the Anthroposophical Movement in Relationship to the Anthroposophical Society. A Stimulus to Self-Contemplation

CW 259   The Year of Destiny 1923 in the History of the Anthroposophical Society. From the Burning of the Goetheanum to the Christmas Conference

CW 260   The Christmas Conference for the Founding of the General Anthroposophical Society

CW 260a   The Constitution of the General Anthroposophical Society and the School for Spiritual Science. The Rebuilding of the Goetheanum

CW 261   Our Dead. Addresses, Words of Remembrance, and Meditative Verses, 1906–1924

CW 262   Rudolf Steiner and Marie Steiner-von Sivers: Correspondence and Documents, 1901–1925

CW 263/1   Rudolf Steiner and Edith Maryon: Correspondence: Letters, Verses, Sketches, 1912–1924

CW 264   On the History and the Contents of the First Section of the Esoteric School from 1904 to 1914. Letters, Newsletters, Documents, Lectures

CW 265   On the History and from the Contents of the Ritual-Knowledge Section of the Esoteric School from 1904 to 1914. Documents, and Lectures from the Years 1906 to 1914, as Well as on New Approaches to Ritual-Knowledge Work in the Years 1921–1924

CW 266/1   From the Contents of the Esoteric Lessons. Volume 1: 1904–
              1909. Notes from Memory of Participants. Meditation texts from
              the notes of Rudolf Steiner
CW 266/2   From the Contents of the Esoteric Lessons. Volume 2: 1910–
              1912. Notes from Memory of Participants
CW 266/3   From the Contents of the Esoteric Lessons. Volume 3: 1913, 1914
              and 1920–1923. Notes from Memory of Participants. Meditation
              texts from the notes of Rudolf Steiner
CW 267   Soul-Exercises: Vol. 1: Exercises with Word and Image Medita-
              tions for the Methodological Development of Higher Powers of
              Knowledge, 1904–1924
CW 268   Soul-Exercises: Vol. 2: Mantric Verses, 1903–1925
CW 269   Ritual Texts for the Celebration of the Free Christian Religious
              Instruction. The Collected Verses for Teachers and Students of the
              Waldorf School
CW 270   Esoteric Instructions for the First Class of the School for Spiritual
              Science at the Goetheanum 1924, 4 Volumes
CW 271   Art and Knowledge of Art. Foundations of a New Aesthetic
CW 272   Spiritual-Scientific Commentary on Goethe's 'Faust' in Two
              Volumes. Vol. 1: Faust, the Striving Human Being
CW 273   Spiritual-Scientific Commentary on Goethe's 'Faust' in Two
              Volumes. Vol. 2: The Faust-Problem
CW 274   Addresses for the Christmas Plays from the Old Folk Traditions
CW 275   Art in the Light of Mystery-Wisdom
CW 276   The Artistic in Its Mission in the World. The Genius of Language.
              The World of Self-Revealing Radiant Appearances—Anthro-
              posophy and Art. Anthroposophy and Poetry
CW 277   Eurythmy. The Revelation of the Speaking Soul
CW 277a   The Origin and Development of Eurythmy
CW 278   Eurythmy as Visible Song
CW 279   Eurythmy as Visible Speech
CW 280   The Method and Nature of Speech Formation
CW 281   The Art of Recitation and Declamation
CW 282   Speech Formation and Dramatic Art
CW 283   The Nature of Things Musical and the Experience of Tone in the
              Human Being
CW 284/285   Images of Occult Seals and Pillars. The Munich Congress of
              Whitsun 1907 and Its Consequences
CW 286   Paths to a New Style of Architecture. 'And the Building Becomes
              Human'
CW 287   The Building at Dornach as a Symbol of Historical Becoming and
              an Artistic Transformation Impulse
CW 288   Style-Forms in the Living Organic
CW 289   The Building-Idea of the Goetheanum: Lectures with Slides from
              the Years 1920–1921
CW 290   The Building-Idea of the Goetheanum: Lectures with Slides from
              the Years 1920–1921

CW 291   The Nature of Colors

CW 291a   Knowledge of Colors. Supplementary Volume to 'The Nature of Colors'

CW 292   Art History as Image of Inner Spiritual Impulses

CW 293   General Knowledge of the Human Being as the Foundation of Pedagogy

CW 294   The Art of Education, Methodology and Didactics

CW 295   The Art of Education: Seminar Discussions and Lectures on Lesson Planning

CW 296   The Question of Education as a Social Question

CW 297   The Idea and Practice of the Waldorf School

CW 297a   Education for Life: Self-Education and the Practice of Pedagogy

CW 298   Rudolf Steiner in the Waldorf School

CW 299   Spiritual-Scientific Observations on Speech

CW 300a   Conferences with the Teachers of the Free Waldorf School in Stuttgart, 1919 to 1924, in 3 Volumes, Vol. 1

CW 300b   Conferences with the Teachers of the Free Waldorf School in Stuttgart, 1919 to 1924, in 3 Volumes, Vol. 2

CW 300c   Conferences with the Teachers of the Free Waldorf School in Stuttgart, 1919 to 1924, in 3 Volumes, Vol. 3

CW 301   The Renewal of Pedagogical-Didactical Art through Spiritual Science

CW 302   Knowledge of the Human Being and the Forming of Class Lessons

CW 302a   Education and Teaching from a Knowledge of the Human Being

CW 303   The Healthy Development of the Human Being

CW 304   Methods of Education and Teaching Based on Anthroposophy

CW 304a   Anthroposophical Knowledge of the Human Being and Pedagogy

CW 305   The Soul-Spiritual Foundational Forces of the Art of Education. Spiritual Values in Education and Social Life

CW 306   Pedagogical Praxis from the Viewpoint of a Spiritual-Scientific Knowledge of the Human Being. The Education of the Child and Young Human Beings

CW 307   The Spiritual Life of the Present and Education

CW 308   The Method of Teaching and the Life-Requirements for Teaching

CW 309   Anthroposophical Pedagogy and Its Prerequisites

CW 310   The Pedagogical Value of a Knowledge of the Human Being and the Cultural Value of Pedagogy

CW 311   The Art of Education from an Understanding of the Being of Humanity

CW 312   Spiritual Science and Medicine

CW 313   Spiritual-Scientific Viewpoints on Therapy

CW 314   Physiology and Therapy Based on Spiritual Science

CW 315   Curative Eurythmy

CW 316   Meditative Observations and Instructions for a Deepening of the Art of Healing

CW 317   The Curative Education Course

CW 318	The Working Together of Doctors and Pastors
CW 319	Anthroposophical Knowledge of the Human Being and Medicine
CW 320	Spiritual-Scientific Impulses for the Development of Physics 1: The First Natural-Scientific Course: Light, Color, Tone, Mass, Electricity, Magnetism
CW 321	Spiritual-Scientific Impulses for the Development of Physics 2: The Second Natural-Scientific Course: Warmth at the Border of Positive and Negative Materiality
CW 322	The Borders of the Knowledge of Nature
CW 323	The Relationship of the various Natural-Scientific Fields to Astronomy
CW 324	Nature Observation, Mathematics, and Scientific Experimentation and Results from the Viewpoint of Anthroposophy
CW 324a	The Fourth Dimension in Mathematics and Reality
CW 325	Natural Science and the World-Historical Development of Humanity since Ancient Times
CW 326	The Moment of the Coming Into Being of Natural Science in World History and Its Development Since Then
CW 327	Spiritual-Scientific Foundations for Success in Farming. The Agricultural Course
CW 328	The Social Question
CW 329	The Liberation of the Human Being as the Foundation for a New Social Form
CW 330	The Renewal of the Social Organism
CW 331	Work-Council and Socialization
CW 332	The Alliance for Threefolding and the Total Reform of Society. The Council on Culture and the Liberation of the Spiritual Life
CW 332a	The Social Future
CW 333	Freedom of Thought and Social Forces
CW 334	From the Unified State to the Threefold Social Organism
CW 335	The Crisis of the Present and the Path to Healthy Thinking
CW 336	The Great Questions of the Times and Anthroposophical Spiritual Knowledge
CW 337a	Social Ideas, Social Reality, Social Practice, Vol. 1: Question-and-Answer Evenings and Study Evenings of the Alliance for the Threefold Social Organism in Stuttgart, 1919–1920
CW 337b	Social Ideas, Social Realities, Social Practice, Vol. 2: Discussion Evenings of the Swiss Alliance for the Threefold Social Organism
CW 338	How Does One Work on Behalf of the Impulse for the Threefold Social Organism?
CW 339	Anthroposophy, Threefold Social Organism, and the Art of Public Speaking
CW 340	The National-Economics Course. The Tasks of a New Science of Economics, Volume 1
CW 341	The National-Economics Seminar. The Tasks of a New Science of Economics, Volume 2

CW 342 Lectures and Courses on Christian Religious Work, Vol. 1: Anthroposophical Foundations for a Renewed Christian Religious Working

CW 343 Lectures and Courses on Christian Religious Work, Vol. 2: Spiritual Knowledge—Religious Feeling—Cultic Doing

CW 344 Lectures and Courses on Christian Religious Work, Vol. 3: Lectures at the Founding of the Christian Community

CW 345 Lectures and Courses on Christian Religious Work, Vol. 4: Concerning the Nature of the Working Word

CW 346 Lectures and Courses on Christian Religious Work, Vol. 5: The Apocalypse and the Work of the Priest

CW 347 The Knowledge of the Nature of the Human Being According to Body, Soul and Spirit. On Earlier Conditions of the Earth

CW 348 On Health and Illness. Foundations of a Spiritual-Scientific Doctrine of the Senses

CW 349 On the Life of the Human Being and of the Earth. On the Nature of Christianity

CW 350 Rhythms in the Cosmos and in the Human Being. How Does One Come To See the Spiritual World?

CW 351 The Human Being and the World. The Influence of the Spirit in Nature. On the Nature of Bees

CW 352 Nature and the Human Being Observed Spiritual-Scientifically

CW 353 The History of Humanity and the World-Views of the Folk Cultures

CW 354 The Creation of the World and the Human Being. Life on Earth and the Influence of the Stars

SIGNIFICANT EVENTS IN THE LIFE OF
RUDOLF STEINER

1829:   June 23: birth of Johann Steiner (1829–1910)—Rudolf Steiner's father—in Geras, Lower Austria.

1834:   May 8: birth of Franciska Blie (1834–1918)—Rudolf Steiner's mother—in Horn, Lower Austria. 'My father and mother were both children of the glorious Lower Austrian forest district north of the Danube.'

1860:   May 16: marriage of Johann Steiner and Franciska Blie.

1861:   February 25: birth of *Rudolf Joseph Lorenz Steiner* in Kraljevec, Croatia, near the border with Hungary, where Johann Steiner works as a telegrapher for the South Austria Railroad. Rudolf Steiner is baptized two days later, February 27, the date usually given as his birthday.

1862:   Summer: the family moves to Mödling, Lower Austria.

1863:   The family moves to Pottschach, Lower Austria, near the Styrian border, where Johann Steiner becomes stationmaster. 'The view stretched to the mountains ... majestic peaks in the distance and the sweet charm of nature in the immediate surroundings.'

1864:   November 15: birth of Rudolf Steiner's sister, Leopoldine (d. November 1, 1927). She will become a seamstress and live with her parents for the rest of her life.

1866:   July 28: birth of Rudolf Steiner's deaf-mute brother, Gustav (d. May 1, 1941).

1867:   Rudolf Steiner enters the village school. Following a disagreement between his father and the schoolmaster, whose wife falsely accused the boy of causing a commotion, Rudolf Steiner is taken out of school and taught at home.

1868:   A critical experience. Unknown to the family, an aunt dies in a distant town. Sitting in the station waiting room, Rudolf Steiner sees her 'form,' which speaks to him, asking for help. 'Beginning with this experience, a new soul life began in the boy, one in which not only the outer trees and mountains spoke to him, but also the worlds that lay behind them. From this moment on, the boy began to live with the spirits of nature ...'

1869:   The family moves to the peaceful, rural village of Neudorfl, near Wiener-Neustadt in present-day Austria. Rudolf Steiner attends the village school. Because of the 'unorthodoxy' of his writing and spelling, he has to do 'extra lessons.'

1870:   Through a book lent to him by his tutor, he discovers geometry: 'To grasp something purely in the spirit brought me inner happiness. I know that I first learned happiness through geometry.' The same tutor allows him to draw, while other students still struggle with their reading and writing. 'An artistic element' thus enters his education.

1871: Though his parents are not religious, Rudolf Steiner becomes a 'church child,' a favorite of the priest, who was 'an exceptional character.' 'Up to the age of ten or eleven, among those I came to know, he was far and away the most significant.' Among other things, he introduces Steiner to Copernican, heliocentric cosmology. As an altar boy, Rudolf Steiner serves at Masses, funerals, and Corpus Christi processions. At year's end, after an incident in which he escapes a thrashing, his father forbids him to go to church.

1872: Rudolf Steiner transfers to grammar school in Wiener-Neustadt, a five-mile walk from home, which must be done in all weathers.

1873–75: Through his teachers and on his own, Rudolf Steiner has many wonderful experiences with science and mathematics. Outside school, he teaches himself analytic geometry, trigonometry, differential equations, and calculus.

1876: Rudolf Steiner begins tutoring other students. He learns bookbinding from his father. He also teaches himself stenography.

1877: Rudolf Steiner discovers Kant's *Critique of Pure Reason*, which he reads and rereads. He also discovers and reads von Rotteck's *World History*.

1878: He studies extensively in contemporary psychology and philosophy.

1879: Rudolf Steiner graduates from high school with honors. His father is transferred to Inzersdorf, near Vienna. He uses his first visit to Vienna 'to purchase a great number of philosophy books'—Kant, Fichte, Schelling, and Hegel, as well as numerous histories of philosophy. His aim: to find a path from the 'I' to nature.

October 1879–1883: Rudolf Steiner attends the Technical College in Vienna—to study mathematics, chemistry, physics, mineralogy, botany, zoology, biology, geology, and mechanics—with a scholarship. He also attends lectures in history and literature, while avidly reading philosophy on his own. His two favorite professors are Karl Julius Schröer (German language and literature) and Edmund Reitlinger (physics). He also audits lectures by Robert Zimmerman on aesthetics and Franz Brentano on philosophy. During this year he begins his friendship with Moritz Zitter (1861–1921), who will help support him financially when he is in Berlin.

1880: Rudolf Steiner attends lectures on Schiller and Goethe by Karl Julius Schröer, who becomes his mentor. Also 'through a remarkable combination of circumstances,' he meets Felix Koguzki, a 'herb gatherer' and healer, who could 'see deeply into the secrets of nature.' Rudolf Steiner will meet and study with this 'emissary of the Master' throughout his time in Vienna.

1881: January: '... I didn't sleep a wink. I was busy with philosophical problems until about 12:30 a.m. Then, finally, I threw myself down on my couch. All my striving during the previous year had been to research whether the following statement by Schelling was true or not: *Within everyone dwells a secret, marvelous capacity to draw back from the stream of time—out of the self clothed in all that comes to us from outside—into our innermost being and there, in the immutable form of the Eternal, to look into ourselves.* I believe, and I am still quite certain of it, that I discovered this capacity in myself; I had long had an inkling of it. Now the whole of idealist philosophy stood before me in modified form. What's a sleepless night compared to that!'

Rudolf Steiner begins communicating with leading thinkers of the day, who send him books in return, which he reads eagerly.

July: 'I am not one of those who dives into the day like an animal in human form. I pursue a quite specific goal, an idealistic aim—knowledge of the truth! This cannot be done offhandedly. It requires the greatest striving in the world, free of all egotism, and equally of all resignation.'

August: Steiner puts down on paper for the first time thoughts for a 'Philosophy of Freedom.' 'The striving for the absolute: this human yearning is freedom.' He also seeks to outline a 'peasant philosophy,' describing what the worldview of a 'peasant'—one who lives close to the earth and the old ways—really is.

1881–1882: Felix Koguzki, the herb gatherer, reveals himself to be the envoy of another, higher initiatory personality, who instructs Rudolf Steiner to penetrate Fichte's philosophy and to master modern scientific thinking as a preparation for right entry into the spirit. This 'Master' also teaches him the double (evolutionary and involutionary) nature of time.

1882:   Through the offices of Karl Julius Schröer, Rudolf Steiner is asked by Joseph Kurschner to edit Goethe's scientific works for the *Deutschen National-Literatur* edition. He writes 'A Possible Critique of Atomistic Concepts' and sends it to Friedrich Theodore Vischer.

1883:   Rudolf Steiner completes his college studies and begins work on the Goethe project.

1884:   First volume of Goethe's *Scientific Writings* (CW 1) appears (March). He lectures on Goethe and Lessing, and Goethe's approach to science. In July, he enters the household of Ladislaus and Pauline Specht as tutor to the four Specht boys. He will live there until 1890. At this time, he meets Josef Breuer (1842–1925), the coauthor with Sigmund Freud of *Studies in Hysteria*, who is the Specht family doctor.

1885:   While continuing to edit Goethe's writings, Rudolf Steiner reads deeply in contemporary philosophy (Edouard von Hartmann, Johannes Volkelt, and Richard Wahle, among others).

1886:   May: Rudolf Steiner sends Kurschner the manuscript of *Outlines of Goethe's Theory of Knowledge* (CW 2), which appears in October, and which he sends out widely. He also meets the poet Marie Eugenie Delle Grazie and writes 'Nature and Our Ideals' for her. He attends her salon, where he meets many priests, theologians, and philosophers, who will become his friends. Meanwhile, the director of the Goethe Archive in Weimar requests his collaboration with the *Sophien* edition of Goethe's works, particularly the writings on color.

1887:   At the beginning of the year, Rudolf Steiner is very sick. As the year progresses and his health improves, he becomes increasingly 'a man of letters,' lecturing, writing essays, and taking part in Austrian cultural life. In August–September, the second volume of Goethe's *Scientific Writings* appears.

1888: January–July: Rudolf Steiner assumes editorship of the 'German Weekly' (*Deutsche Wochenschrift*). He begins lecturing more intensively, giving, for example, a lecture titled 'Goethe as Father of a New Aesthetics.' He meets and becomes soul friends with Friedrich Eckstein (1861–1939), a vegetarian, philosopher of symbolism, alchemist, and musician, who will introduce him to various spiritual currents (including Theosophy) and with whom he will meditate and interpret esoteric and alchemical texts.

1889: Rudolf Steiner first reads Nietzsche (*Beyond Good and Evil*). He encounters Theosophy again and learns of Madame Blavatsky in the Theosophical circle around Marie Lang (1858–1934). Here he also meets well-known figures of Austrian life, as well as esoteric figures like the occultist Franz Hartman and Karl Leinigen-Billigen (translator of C.G. Harrison's *The Transcendental Universe*). During this period, Steiner first reads A.P. Sinnett's *Esoteric Buddhism* and Mabel Collins's *Light on the Path*. He also begins traveling, visiting Budapest, Weimar, and Berlin (where he meets philosopher Edouard von Hartmann).

1890: Rudolf Steiner finishes volume 3 of Goethe's scientific writings. He begins his doctoral dissertation, which will become *Truth and Science* (CW 3). He also meets the poet and feminist Rosa Mayreder (1858–1938), with whom he can exchange his most intimate thoughts. In September, Rudolf Steiner moves to Weimar to work in the Goethe-Schiller Archive.

1891: Volume 3 of the Kurschner edition of Goethe appears. Meanwhile, Rudolf Steiner edits Goethe's studies in mineralogy and scientific writings for the *Sophien* edition. He meets Ludwig Laistner of the Cotta Publishing Company, who asks for a book on the basic question of metaphysics. From this will result, ultimately, *The Philosophy of Freedom* (CW 4), which will be published not by Cotta but by Emil Felber. In October, Rudolf Steiner takes the oral exam for a doctorate in philosophy, mathematics, and mechanics at Rostock University, receiving his doctorate on the twenty-sixth. In November, he gives his first lecture on Goethe's 'Fairy Tale' in Vienna.

1892: Rudolf Steiner continues work at the Goethe-Schiller Archive and on his *Philosophy of Freedom*. *Truth and Science*, his doctoral dissertation, is published. Steiner undertakes to write introductions to books on Schopenhauer and Jean Paul for Cotta. At year's end, he finds lodging with Anna Eunike, née Schulz (1853–1911), a widow with four daughters and a son. He also develops a friendship with Otto Erich Hartleben (1864–1905) with whom he shares literary interests.

1893: Rudolf Steiner begins his habit of producing many reviews and articles. In March, he gives a lecture titled 'Hypnotism, with Reference to Spiritism.' In September, volume 4 of the Kurschner edition is completed. In November, *The Philosophy of Freedom* appears. This year, too, he meets John Henry Mackay (1864–1933), the anarchist, and Max Stirner, a scholar and biographer.

1894: Rudolf Steiner meets Elisabeth Förster Nietzsche, the philosopher's sister, and begins to read Nietzsche in earnest, beginning with the as yet unpublished *Antichrist*. He also meets Ernst Haeckel (1834–1919). In the fall, he begins to write *Nietzsche, A Fighter against His Time* (CW 5).

1895: May, *Nietzsche, A Fighter against His Time* appears.

1896: January 22: Rudolf Steiner sees Friedrich Nietzsche for the first and only time. Moves between the Nietzsche and the Goethe-Schiller Archives, where he completes his work before year's end. He falls out with Elisabeth Förster Nietzsche, thus ending his association with the Nietzsche Archive.

1897: Rudolf Steiner finishes the manuscript of *Goethe's Worldview* (CW 6). He moves to Berlin with Anna Eunike and begins editorship of the *Magazin fur Literatur*. From now on, Steiner will write countless reviews, literary and philosophical articles, and so on. He begins lecturing at the 'Free Literary Society.' In September, he attends the Zionist Congress in Basel. He sides with Dreyfus in the Dreyfus affair.

1898: Rudolf Steiner is very active as an editor in the political, artistic, and theatrical life of Berlin. He becomes friendly with John Henry Mackay and poet Ludwig Jacobowski (1868–1900). He joins Jacobowski's circle of writers, artists, and scientists—'The Coming Ones' (*Die Kommenden*)—and contributes lectures to the group until 1903. He also lectures at the 'League for College Pedagogy.' He writes an article for Goethe's sesquicentennial, 'Goethe's Secret Revelation,' on the 'Fairy Tale of the Green Snake and the Beautiful Lily.'

1898–99: 'This was a trying time for my soul as I looked at Christianity. . . . I was able to progress only by contemplating, by means of spiritual perception, the evolution of Christianity. . . . Conscious knowledge of real Christianity began to dawn in me around the turn of the century. This seed continued to develop. My soul trial occurred shortly before the beginning of the twentieth century. It was decisive for my soul's development that I stood spiritually before the Mystery of Golgotha in a deep and solemn celebration of knowledge.'

1899: Rudolf Steiner begins teaching and giving lectures and lecture cycles at the Workers' College, founded by Wilhelm Liebknecht (1826–1900). He will continue to do so until 1904. Writes: *Literature and Spiritual Life in the Nineteenth Century; Individualism in Philosophy; Haeckel and His Opponents; Poetry in the Present;* and begins what will become (fifteen years later) *The Riddles of Philosophy* (CW 18). He also meets many artists and writers, including Käthe Kollwitz, Stefan Zweig, and Rainer Maria Rilke. On October 31, he marries Anna Eunike.

1900: 'I thought that the turn of the century must bring humanity a new light. It seemed to me that the separation of human thinking and willing from the spirit had peaked. A turn or reversal of direction in human evolution seemed to me a necessity.' Rudolf Steiner finishes *World and Life Views in the Nineteenth Century* (the second part of what will become *The Riddles of Philosophy*) and dedicates it to Ernst Haeckel. It is published in March. He continues lecturing at *Die Kommenden*, whose leadership he assumes after the death of Jacobowski. Also, he gives the Gutenberg Jubilee lecture before 7,000 typesetters and printers. In September, Rudolf Steiner is invited by Count and Countess Brockdorff to lecture in the Theosophical Library. His first lecture is on Nietzsche. His second lecture is titled 'Goethe's Secret Revelation.' October 6, he begins a lecture cycle on the mystics that will become *Mystics after Modernism* (CW 7). November-December: 'Marie von Sivers appears in the audience. . . .' Also in November, Steiner gives his first lecture at the Giordano Bruno Bund (where he will continue to lecture until May, 1905). He speaks on Bruno and modern Rome, focusing on the importance of the philosophy of Thomas Aquinas as monism.

1901· In continual financial straits, Rudolf Steiner's early friends Moritz Zitter and Rosa Mayreder help support him. In October, he begins the lecture cycle *Christianity as Mystical Fact* (CW 8) at the Theosophical Library. In November, he gives his first 'Theosophical lecture' on Goethe's 'Fairy Tale' in Hamburg at the invitation of Wilhelm Hubbe-Schleiden. He also attends a gathering to celebrate the founding of the Theosophical Society at Count and Countess Brockdorff's. He gives a lecture cycle, 'From Buddha to Christ,' for the circle of the *Kommenden*. November 17, Marie von Sivers asks Rudolf Steiner if Theosophy needs a Western-Christian spiritual movement (to complement Theosophy's Eastern emphasis). 'The question was posed. Now, following spiritual laws, I could begin to give an answer. . . .' In December, Rudolf Steiner writes his first article for a Theosophical publication. At year's end, the Brockdorffs and possibly Wilhelm Hubbe-Schleiden ask Rudolf Steiner to join the Theosophical Society and undertake the leadership of the German section. Rudolf Steiner agrees, on the condition that Marie von Sivers (then in Italy) work with him.

1902: Beginning in January, Rudolf Steiner attends the opening of the Workers' School in Spandau with Rosa Luxemberg (1870–1919). January 17, Rudolf Steiner joins the Theosophical Society. In April, he is asked to become general secretary of the German Section of the Theosophical Society, and works on preparations for its founding. In July, he visits London for a Theosophical congress. He meets Bertram Keightly, G.R.S. Mead, A.P. Sinnett, and Annie Besant, among others. In September, *Christianity as Mystical Fact* appears. In October, Rudolf Steiner gives his first public lecture on Theosophy ('Monism and Theosophy') to about three hundred people at the Giordano Bruno Bund. On October 19–21, the German Section of the Theosophical Society has its first meeting; Rudolf Steiner is the general secretary, and Annie Besant attends. Steiner lectures on practical karma studies. On October 23, Annie Besant inducts Rudolf Steiner into the Esoteric School of the Theosophical Society. On October 25, Steiner begins a weekly series of lectures: 'The Field of Theosophy.' During this year, Rudolf Steiner also first meets Ita Wegman (1876–1943), who will become his close collaborator in his final years.

1903: Rudolf Steiner holds about 300 lectures and seminars. In May, the first issue of the periodical *Luzifer* appears. In June, Rudolf Steiner visits

London for the first meeting of the Federation of the European Sections of the Theosophical Society, where he meets Colonel Olcott. He begins to write *Theosophy* (CW 9).

1904: Rudolf Steiner continues lecturing at the Workers' College and elsewhere (about 90 lectures), while lecturing intensively all over Germany among Theosophists (about 140 lectures). In February, he meets Carl Unger (1878–1929), who will become a member of the board of the Anthroposophical Society (1913). In March, he meets Michael Bauer (1871–1929), a Christian mystic, who will also be on the board. In May, *Theosophy* appears, with the dedication: 'To the spirit of Giordano Bruno.' Rudolf Steiner and Marie von Sivers visit London for meetings with Annie Besant. June: Rudolf Steiner and Marie von Sivers attend the meeting of the Federation of European Sections of the Theosophical Society in Amsterdam. In July, Steiner begins the articles in *Luzifer-Gnosis* that will become *How to Know Higher Worlds* (CW 10) and *Cosmic Memory* (CW 11). In September, Annie Besant visits Germany. In December, Steiner lectures on Freemasonry. He mentions the High Grade Masonry derived from John Yarker and represented by Theodore Reuss and Karl Kellner as a blank slate 'into which a good image could be placed.'

1905: This year, Steiner ends his non-Theosophical lecturing activity. Supported by Marie von Sivers, his Theosophical lecturing—both in public and in the Theosophical Society—increases significantly: 'The German Theosophical Movement is of exceptional importance.' Steiner recommends reading, among others, Fichte, Jacob Boehme, and Angelus Silesius. He begins to introduce Christian themes into Theosophy. He also begins to work with doctors (Felix Peipers and Ludwig Noll). In July, he is in London for the Federation of European Sections, where he attends a lecture by Annie Besant: 'I have seldom seen Mrs. Besant speak in so inward and heartfelt a manner....' 'Through Mrs. Besant I have found the way to H.P. Blavatsky.' September to October, he gives a course of thirty-one lectures for a small group of esoteric students. In October, the annual meeting of the German Section of the Theosophical Society, which still remains very small, takes place. Rudolf Steiner reports membership has risen from 121 to 377 members. In November, seeking to establish esoteric 'continuity,' Rudolf Steiner and Marie von Sivers participate in a 'Memphis-Misraim' Masonic ceremony. They pay forty-five marks for membership. 'Yesterday, you saw how little remains of former esoteric institutions.' 'We are dealing only with a "framework"... for the present, nothing lies behind it. The occult powers have completely withdrawn.'

1906: Expansion of Theosophical work. Rudolf Steiner gives about 245 lectures, only 44 of which take place in Berlin. Cycles are given in Paris, Leipzig, Stuttgart, and Munich. Esoteric work also intensifies. Rudolf Steiner begins writing *An Outline of Esoteric Science* (CW 13). In January, Rudolf Steiner receives permission (a patent) from the Great Orient of the Scottish A & A Thirty-Three Degree Rite of the Order of the Ancient

Freemasons of the Memphis-Misraim Rite to direct a chapter under the name 'Mystica Aeterna.' This will become the 'Cognitive-Ritual Section' (also called 'Misraim Service') of the Esoteric School. (See: *Freemasonry and Ritual Work: The Misraim Service*, CW 265). During this time, Steiner also meets Albert Schweitzer. In May, he is in Paris, where he visits Edouard Schuré. Many Russians attend his lectures (including Konstantin Balmont, Dimitri Mereszkovski, Zinaida Hippius, and Maximilian Woloshin). He attends the General Meeting of the European Federation of the Theosophical Society, at which Col. Olcott is present for the last time. He spends the year's end in Venice and Rome, where he writes and works on his translation of H.P. Blavatsky's *Key to Theosophy*.

1907: Further expansion of the German Theosophical Movement according to the Rosicrucian directive to 'introduce spirit into the world'—in education, in social questions, in art, and in science. In February, Col. Olcott dies in Adyar. Before he dies, Olcott indicates that 'the Masters' wish Annie Besant to succeed him: much politicking ensues. Rudolf Steiner supports Besant's candidacy. April-May: preparations for the Congress of the Federation of European Sections of the Theosophical Society—the great, watershed Whitsun 'Munich Congress,' attended by Annie Besant and others. Steiner decides to separate Eastern and Western (Christian-Rosicrucian) esoteric schools. He takes his esoteric school out of the Theosophical Society (Besant and Rudolf Steiner are 'in harmony' on this). Steiner makes his first lecture tours to Austria and Hungary. That summer, he is in Italy. In September, he visits Edouard Schuré, who will write the introduction to the French edition of *Christianity as Mystical Fact* in Barr, Alsace. Rudolf Steiner writes the autobiographical statement known as the 'Barr Document.' In *Luzifer-Gnosis*, 'The Education of the Child' appears.

1908: The movement grows (membership: 1,150). Lecturing expands. Steiner makes his first extended lecture tour to Holland and Scandinavia, as well as visits to Naples and Sicily. Themes: St. John's Gospel, the Apocalypse, Egypt, science, philosophy, and logic. *Luzifer-Gnosis* ceases publication. In Berlin, Marie von Sivers (with Johanna Mücke (1864–1949) forms the *Philosophisch-Theosophisch* (after 1915 *Philosophisch-Anthroposophisch*) *Verlag* to publish Steiner's work. Steiner gives lecture cycles titled *The Gospel of St. John* (CW 103) and *The Apocalypse* (104).

1909: *An Outline of Esoteric Science* appears. Lecturing and travel continues. Rudolf Steiner's spiritual research expands to include the polarity of Lucifer and Ahriman; the work of great individualities in history; the Maitreya Buddha and the Bodhisattvas; spiritual economy (CW 109); the work of the spiritual hierarchies in heaven and on earth (CW 110). He also deepens and intensifies his research into the Gospels, giving lectures on the Gospel of St. Luke (CW 114) with the first mention of two Jesus children. Meets and becomes friends with Christian Morgenstern (1871–1914). In April, he lays the foundation stone for the Malsch model—the building that will lead to the first Goetheanum. In May, the International Congress of the Federation of European Sections of the

Theosophical Society takes place in Budapest. Rudolf Steiner receives the Subba Row medal for *How to Know Higher Worlds*. During this time, Charles W. Leadbeater discovers Jiddu Krishnamurti (1895–1986) and proclaims him the future 'world teacher,' the bearer of the Maitreya Buddha and the 'reappearing Christ.' In October, Steiner delivers seminal lectures on 'anthroposophy,' which he will try, unsuccessfully, to rework over the next years into the unfinished work, *Anthroposophy (A Fragment)* (CW 45).

1910: New themes: *The Reappearance of Christ in the Etheric* (CW 118); *The Fifth Gospel; The Mission of Folk Souls* (CW 121); *Occult History* (CW 126); the evolving development of etheric cognitive capacities. Rudolf Steiner continues his Gospel research with *The Gospel of St. Matthew* (CW 123). In January, his father dies. In April, he takes a month-long trip to Italy, including Rome, Monte Cassino, and Sicily. He also visits Scandinavia again. July–August, he writes the first mystery drama, *The Portal of Initiation* (CW 14). In November, he gives 'psychosophy' lectures. In December, he submits 'On the Psychological Foundations and Epistemological Framework of Theosophy' to the International Philosophical Congress in Bologna.

1911: The crisis in the Theosophical Society deepens. In January, 'The Order of the Rising Sun,' which will soon become 'The Order of the Star in the East,' is founded for the coming world teacher, Krishnamurti. At the same time, Marie von Sivers, Rudolf Steiner's coworker, falls ill. Fewer lectures are given, but important new ground is broken. In Prague, in March, Steiner meets Franz Kafka (1883–1924) and Hugo Bergmann (1883-1975). In April, he delivers his paper to the Philosophical Congress. He writes the second mystery drama, *The Soul's Probation* (CW 14). Also, while Marie von Sivers is convalescing, Rudolf Steiner begins work on *Calendar 1912/1913*, which will contain the 'Calendar of the Soul' meditations. On March 19, Anna (Eunike) Steiner dies. In September, Rudolf Steiner visits Einsiedeln, birthplace of Paracelsus. In December, Friedrich Rittelmeyer, future founder of the Christian Community, meets Rudolf Steiner. The *Johannes-Bauverein*, the 'building committee,' which would lead to the first Goetheanum (first planned for Munich), is also founded, and a preliminary committee for the founding of an independent association is created that, in the following year, will become the Anthroposophical Society. Important lecture cycles include *Occult Physiology* (CW 128); *Wonders of the World* (CW 129); *From Jesus to Christ* (CW 131). Other themes: esoteric Christianity; Christian Rosenkreutz; the spiritual guidance of humanity; the sense world and the world of the spirit.

1912: Despite the ongoing, now increasing crisis in the Theosophical Society, much is accomplished: *Calendar 1912/1913* is published; eurythmy is created; both the third mystery drama, *The Guardian of the Threshold* (CW 14) and *A Way of Self-Knowledge* (CW 16) are written. New (or renewed) themes included life between death and rebirth and karma and reincarnation. Other lecture cycles: *Spiritual Beings in the Heavenly Bodies and in the Kingdoms of Nature* (CW 136); *The Human Being in the Light of Occultism, Theosophy, and Philosophy* (CW 137); *The Gospel of St. Mark* (CW 139); and *The Bhagavad Gita and the Epistles of Paul* (CW 142). On May 8, Rudolf Steiner celebrates White Lotus Day, H.P. Blavatsky's death day, which he had faithfully observed for the past decade, for the last time. In August, Rudolf Steiner suggests the 'independent association' be called the 'Anthroposophical Society.' In September, the first eurythmy course takes place. In October, Rudolf Steiner declines recognition of a Theosophical Society lodge dedicated to the Star of the East and decides to expel all Theosophical Society members belonging to the order. Also, with Marie von Sivers, he first visits Dornach, near Basel, Switzerland, and they stand on the hill where the Goetheanum will be built. In November, a Theosophical Society lodge is opened by direct mandate from Adyar (Annie Besant). In December, a meeting of the German section occurs at which it is decided that belonging to the Order of the Star of the East is incompatible with membership in the Theosophical Society. December 28: informal founding of the Anthroposophical Society in Berlin.

1913: Expulsion of the German section from the Theosophical Society. February 2–3: Foundation meeting of the Anthroposophical Society. Board members include: Marie von Sivers, Michael Bauer, and Carl Unger. September 20: Laying of the foundation stone for the *Johannes Bau* (Goetheanum) in Dornach. Building begins immediately. The third mystery drama, *The Soul's Awakening* (CW 14), is completed. Also: *The Threshold of the Spiritual World* (CW 147). Lecture cycles include: *The Bhagavad Gita and the Epistles of Paul* and *The Esoteric Meaning of the Bhagavad Gita* (CW 146), which the Russian philosopher Nikolai Berdyaev attends; *The Mysteries of the East and of Christianity* (CW 144); *The Effects of Esoteric Development* (CW 145); and *The Fifth Gospel* (CW 148). In May, Rudolf Steiner is in London and Paris, where anthroposophical work continues.

1914: Building continues on the *Johannes Bau* (Goetheanum) in Dornach, with artists and coworkers from seventeen nations. The general assembly of the Anthroposophical Society takes place. In May, Rudolf Steiner visits Paris, as well as Chartres Cathedral. June 28: assassination in Sarajevo ('Now the catastrophe has happened!'). August 1: War is declared. Rudolf Steiner returns to Germany from Dornach—he will travel back and forth. He writes the last chapter of *The Riddles of Philosophy*. Lecture cycles include: *Human and Cosmic Thought* (CW 151); *Inner Being of Humanity between Death and a New Birth* (CW 153); *Occult Reading and Occult Hearing* (CW 156). December 24: marriage of Rudolf Steiner and Marie von Sivers.

1915: Building continues. Life after death becomes a major theme, also art. Writes: *Thoughts during a Time of War* (CW 24). Lectures include: *The Secret of Death* (CW 159); *The Uniting of Humanity through the Christ Impulse* (CW 165).

1916: Rudolf Steiner begins work with Edith Maryon (1872–1924) on the sculpture 'The Representative of Humanity' ('The Group'—Christ, Lucifer, and Ahriman). He also works with the alchemist Alexander von Bernus on the quarterly *Das Reich*. He writes *The Riddle of Humanity* (CW 20). Lectures include: *Necessity and Freedom in World History and Human Action* (CW 166); *Past and Present in the Human Spirit* (CW 167); *The Karma of Vocation* (CW 172); *The Karma of Untruthfulness* (CW 173).

1917: Russian Revolution. The U.S. enters the war. Building continues. Rudolf Steiner delineates the idea of the 'threefold nature of the human being' (in a public lecture March 15) and the 'threefold nature of the social organism' (hammered out in May-June with the help of Otto von Lerchenfeld and Ludwig Polzer-Hoditz in the form of two documents titled *Memoranda*, which were distributed in high places). August–September: Rudolf Steiner writes *The Riddles of the Soul* (CW 20). Also: commentary on 'The Chemical Wedding of Christian Rosenkreutz' for Alexander Bernus (*Das Reich*). Lectures include: *The Karma of Materialism* (CW 176); *The Spiritual Background of the Outer World: The Fall of the Spirits of Darkness* (CW 177).

1918: March 18: peace treaty of Brest-Litovsk—'Now everything will truly enter chaos! What is needed is cultural renewal.' June: Rudolf Steiner visits Karlstein (Grail) Castle outside Prague. Lecture cycle: *From Symptom to Reality in Modern History* (CW 185). In mid-November, Emil Molt, of the Waldorf-Astoria Cigarette Company, has the idea of founding a school for his workers' children.

1919: Focus on the threefold social organism: tireless travel, countless lectures, meetings, and publications. At the same time, a new public stage of Anthroposophy emerges as cultural renewal begins. The coming years will see initiatives in pedagogy, medicine, pharmacology, and agriculture. January 27: threefold meeting: ' We must first of all, with the money we have, found free schools that can bring people what they need.' February: first public eurythmy performance in Zurich. Also: 'Appeal to the German People' (CW 24), circulated March 6 as a newspaper insert. In April, *Towards Social Renewal* (CW 23) appears— 'perhaps the most widely read of all books on politics appearing since the war.' Rudolf Steiner is asked to undertake the 'direction and leadership' of the school founded by the Waldorf-Astoria Company. Rudolf Steiner begins to talk about the 'renewal' of education. May 30: a building is selected and purchased for the future Waldorf School. August–September, Rudolf Steiner gives a lecture course for Waldorf teachers, *The Foundations of Human Experience (Study of Man)* (CW 293). September 7: Opening of the first Waldorf School. December (into January): first science course, the *Light Course* (CW 320).

1920: The Waldorf School flourishes. New threefold initiatives. Founding of limited companies *Der Kommende Tag* and *Futurum A.G.* to infuse spiritual values into the economic realm. Rudolf Steiner also focuses on the sciences. Lectures: *Introducing Anthroposophical Medicine* (CW 312); *The Warmth Course* (CW 321); *The Boundaries of Natural Science* (CW 322); *The Redemption of Thinking* (CW 74). February: Johannes Werner

Klein—later a cofounder of the Christian Community—asks Rudolf Steiner about the possibility of a 'religious renewal,' a 'Johannine church.' In March, Rudolf Steiner gives the first course for doctors and medical students. In April, a divinity student asks Rudolf Steiner a second time about the possibility of religious renewal. September 27–October 16: anthroposophical 'university course.' December: lectures titled *The Search for the New Isis* (CW 202).

1921:   Rudolf Steiner continues his intensive work on cultural renewal, including the uphill battle for the threefold social order. 'University' arts, scientific, theological, and medical courses include: *The Astronomy Course* (CW 323); *Observation, Mathematics, and Scientific Experiment* (CW 324); the *Second Medical Course* (CW 313); *Color*. In June and September-October, Rudolf Steiner also gives the first two 'priests' courses' (CW 342 and 343). The 'youth movement' gains momentum. Magazines are founded: *Die Drei* (January), and—under the editorship of Albert Steffen (1884–1963)—the weekly, *Das Goetheanum* (August). In February–March, Rudolf Steiner takes his first trip outside Germany since the war (Holland). On April 7, Steiner receives a letter regarding 'religious renewal,' and May 22–23, he agrees to address the question in a practical way. In June, the Klinical-Therapeutic Institute opens in Arlesheim under the direction of Dr. Ita Wegman. In August, the Chemical-Pharmaceutical Laboratory opens in Arlesheim (Oskar Schmiedel and Ita Wegman are directors). The Clinical Therapeutic Institute is inaugurated in Stuttgart (Dr. Ludwig Noll is director); also the Research Laboratory in Dornach (Ehrenfried Pfeiffer and Gunther Wachsmuth are directors). In November–December, Rudolf Steiner visits Norway.

1922:   The first half of the year involves very active public lecturing (thousands attend); in the second half, Rudolf Steiner begins to withdraw and turn toward the Society—'The Society is asleep.' It is 'too weak' to do what is asked of it. The businesses—*Der Kommende Tag* and *Futurum A.G.*—fail. In January, with the help of an agent, Steiner undertakes a twelve-city German lecture tour, accompanied by eurythmy performances. In two weeks he speaks to more than 2,000 people. In April, he gives a 'university course' in The Hague. He also visits England. In June, he is in Vienna for the East–West Congress. In August–September, he is back in England for the Oxford Conference on Education. Returning to Dornach, he gives the lectures *Philosophy, Cosmology, and Religion* (CW 215), and gives the third priests' course (CW 344). On September 16, The Christian Community is founded. In October–November, Steiner is in Holland and England. He also speaks to the youth: *The Youth Course* (CW 217). In December, Steiner gives lectures titled *The Origins of Natural Science* (CW 326), and *Humanity and the World of Stars: The Spiritual Communion of Humanity* (CW 219). December 31: Fire at the Goetheanum, which is destroyed.

1923:   Despite the fire, Rudolf Steiner continues his work unabated. A very hard year. Internal dispersion, dissension, and apathy abound. There is conflict—between old and new visions—within the Society. A wake-up call is needed, and Rudolf Steiner responds with renewed lecturing vitality. His focus: the spiritual context of human life; initiation science; the course of the year; and community building. As a foundation for an artistic school, he creates a series of pastel sketches. Lecture cycles: *The Anthroposophical Movement; Initiation Science* (CW 227) (in England at the Penmaenmawr Summer School); *The Four Seasons and the Archangels* (CW 229); *Harmony of the Creative Word* (CW 230); *The Supersensible Human* (CW 231), given in Holland for the founding of the Dutch society. On November 10, in response to the failed Hitler-Ludendorf putsch in Munich, Steiner closes his Berlin residence and moves the *Philosophisch-Anthroposophisch Verlag* (Press) to Dornach. On December 9, Steiner begins the serialization of his *Autobiography: The Course of My Life* (CW 28) in *Das Goetheanum*. It will continue to appear weekly, without a break, until his death. Late December–early January: Rudolf Steiner re-founds the Anthroposophical Society (about 12,000 members internationally) and takes over its leadership. The new board members are: Marie Steiner, Ita Wegman, Albert Steffen, Elizabeth Vreede, and Guenther Wachsmuth. (See *The Christmas Meeting for the Founding of the General Anthroposophical Society*, CW 260). Accompanying lectures: *Mystery Knowledge and Mystery Centers* (CW 232); *World History in the Light of Anthroposophy* (CW 233). December 25: the Foundation Stone is laid (in the hearts of members) in the form of the 'Foundation Stone Meditation.'

1924:   January 1: having founded the Anthroposophical Society and taken over its leadership, Rudolf Steiner has the task of 'reforming' it. The process begins with a weekly newssheet ('What's Happening in the Anthroposophical Society') in which Rudolf Steiner's 'Letters to Members' and 'Anthroposophical Leading Thoughts' appear (CW 26). The next step is the creation of a new esoteric class, the 'first class' of the 'University of Spiritual Science' (which was to have been followed, had Rudolf Steiner lived longer, by two more advanced classes). Then comes a new language for Anthroposophy—practical, phenomenological, and direct; and Rudolf Steiner creates the model for the second Goetheanum. He begins the series of extensive 'karma' lectures (CW 235–40); and finally, responding to needs, he creates two new initiatives: biodynamic agriculture and curative education. After the middle of the year, rumors begin to circulate regarding Steiner's health. Lectures: January–February, *Anthroposophy* (CW 234); February: *Tone Eurythmy* (CW 278); June: *The Agriculture Course* (CW 327); June–July: *Speech Eurythmy* (CW 279); *Curative Education* (CW 317); August: (England, 'Second International Summer School'), *Initiation Consciousness: True and False Paths in Spiritual Investigation* (CW 243); September: *Pastoral Medicine* (CW 318). On September 26, for the first time, Rudolf Steiner cancels a lecture. On September 28, he gives his last lecture. On September 29, he withdraws to his studio in the carpenter's shop; now he is definitively ill. Cared for by Ita Wegman, he continues working, however, and writing the weekly installments of his *Autobiography* and *Letters to the Members/Leading Thoughts* (CW 26).

1925: Rudolf Steiner, while continuing to work, continues to weaken. He finishes *Extending Practical Medicine* (CW 27) with Ita Wegman. On March 30, around ten in the morning, Rudolf Steiner dies.

INDEX

Abraham, 90, 177
abstinence, 45
abstract/abstraction, 13, 96, 98–99, 123, 184
Achilles, 35
action, logic of, 8
Adam, 88
adversary spiritual beings, 189
Agamemnon, 35
aggression, 57
Ahriman/ahrimanic, 131–139, 189, 193–194, 198
  as Angra Mainyu, 131
  Ahriman as satanic, 194
  ahrimanic beings, 189, 191–194
  in chains, 133, 135
  as the devil, 133
  his fire powers, 134
  his karma, 138–139
Ahriman-Mephistopheles, 134
Ahura Mazda, 108, 131, 196
  as Great Aura, 108, 131
  as sun god, 132
akashic record, 71, 132
alarm, 3
Alberto, Carlo, King, 7
ambition, 143
anatomy, 60, 78, 86
Andromache, 217
angels, 152–153
  angelic, 128
  as sons of life, 152
animal kingdom/animals, xvii, 17–21, 23–25, 30, 45, 54, 56, 63, 81, 94, 107, 111, 114, 124, 128, 130, 132, 192, 195, 206–213, 215, 218, 220–222, 226
  sexual maturity, 221

anthroposophical/anthroposophy, xiii, 1–2, 14–16, 24, 27, 42–43, 52, 54, 60–62, 72, 74, 76–78, 81, 87–88, 95, 98, 103, 107–108, 115, 120, 122–124, 140, 142, 146, 154–157, 159–160, 170–172, 183–186, 188, 199–203, 205–206, 218–219, 223, 231, 234, 236
anthroposophical movement, 11, 14, 47, 60, 102, 144, 200–201, 203
  as wisdom of the spirit, 199
Anthroposophical Society, 234
antimony, 112
antipathy, 40
anxiety, 7, 68, 70–71
Apis culture, 95
Apocalypse, book of, 56, 203
Apollo, 170
Apostles, 178, 180, 200
archangels, 152
  as fire spirits, 152
archetype, 70–71
arrhythmia, 153
ascending/ascent, 38–40
asceticism, 52
Asclepius, rites of, 170
Assyrian, 32–33
astral/astrality, 5–6, 8, 10, 12, 17–21, 23–24, 26, 41–42, 48–50, 63–64, 98, 118, 129, 134, 141, 180, 185–187, 219, 229
  envelope, 219
  forces, 23, 210
  images, 41
  substantiality, 18–19, 23
astral body, 16–17, 20–21, 23, 29, 43, 49–51, 53, 63, 65, 70, 76, 78,

80–81, 84, 91–95, 110–114,
116–118, 120–124, 127–130,
144–150–156, 158–160, 162,
175–187, 190–191, 193, 198,
203, 208–213, 219–222, 229
it contracts, 208–211, 213–214
it expands, 209–211, 213–214
Jesus' replicated, 180–183
rhythmic change, 118, 121–122
as sentient or soul body, 193
seven-day cycle, 145–146
transformed, 187
universal, 117–118
astral plane/world, 2–13, 18–21, 41,
43–45, 51, 110, 129, 174, 180,
209
of evil (lower), 12–13
of goodness, 12–13
astrology/astronomy, 32, 123
Asuras/asuric
(evil ones), 194–195
(good ones), 136
Atlantean/Atlantis, 30–31, 54–55,
102, 107, 109, 122–123,
127–132, 136–137, 139,
150–151, 173, 188–189,
191–194
oracles, 129, 196
post-Atlantean, 31, 54, 102, 132,
136, 173–174, 189, 203
atmospheric phenomena (earth), 130,
139–142
clouds, 130
earthquakes, 125, 138–141
eruptions (volcanic), 138–139
lightning, 4, 130, 138
thunder, 130, 138
water, 134
weather, 132
wind, 132, 134
Augustine of Hippo, 178–179
avatar, 173, 175–177
awareness. See self-awareness

Babylonian, 32–33
bacilli, 95
back-to-nature prophets, 153

balance/balancing, 21–22, 26, 39, 46,
57, 123, 137, 191, 208, 217
counter-balance, 196
beauty, 232
Bedouin, 100
benevolent/benevolence, 5–6, 190, 199
betaine hydrochloride, 80
Bible (Holy), 87–88, 91, 96, 177, 195,
212
birds, 58
black cross, with roses, 41
black magic, 45, 98, 131–132, 135
Blake, William, xv
bliss/blissful, 31–32, 34, 45–46,
50–53, 70–71
accumulated strength, 50
blood, 77–80, 83, 118, 158, 176, 211
circulation, 168
as expression of I nature, 77–78, 80,
158
blossom, 17
bond of attraction, 163–164
bones, 55
boon, 199, 204
botany, 16
Brahma, 202
brain, 52–53, 82, 164, 168, 207,
219–220
breathing, 211–212, 214
Bruno, Giordano, 184
Buddha, 33, 36, 202–203
Buddhi. See Life Spirit (Buddhi)
bull, 56–60
bull-nature, 59–60
bull-race/type, 58–59
burning bush, 97

Calvin, 183
capacities, 207
carbon, 48
Catholic Church, 178, 234
causation, law of, 159
Chaldean, 32–33
Chaldean-Babylonian, 231
change of teeth, 218
chaos/chaotic, 50, 156–157
Charlemagne, 67

child/children, 65, 75, 167, 207–208, 215, 218–220
Chimera, 135
Chiron (centaur), 170
Christ, 27–29, 34, 37, 91, 101, 133, 135, 173, 177–180, 182–183, 185–186, 196–203, 232–233
appeared in underworld, 196
as an avatar, 177, 182, 185
blood of, 183
His blood ran from wounds, 133, 196
Christ event, 197, 232
Christ experience, 232
Christ-less, 196–197
Christ Mystery, 135–136
Christ principle, 177
crucified, 180
descent into hell, 37
I am, 90
I am the I am, 90–91, 196
image of, 179
is the light, 199
as the light of the lodge of the twelve, 200
one who suffered at Golgotha, 101
His primal wisdom, 185
as spirit of the sun, 196
This is my body and this is my blood, 183
as the Word, 233
Christian/Christianity, 28, 87, 91, 100–101, 160, 178–180, 182, 184–187, 199–200, 203
Christian esotericism, 232–234
Christian initiation, 52
Christian Life Spirit, 187
Christian Spirit Self, 187
fire of Christianity, 199
pre-Christian, 35–36, 177
post-Christian, 29, 186
clairvoyance/clairvoyant, 3–4, 18–20, 23, 29, 85, 104, 112, 119, 129, 141, 173, 179–180, 182, 215, 219–220, 223
hindrances, 142
twilight clairvoyance, 32

climatic, 66
clock, humans were as one, 151
clockmaker, 103
Coelenterata phylum, 23
cognition/cognitive, 15, 40, 42, 46, 51, 53, 131, 186
colours, 31, 41–43, 108
astral, 129
communal coexistence, 8
communion, 18
community, members, 22
compassion, 140
compression, 119
concept/conceptual, 5–7, 15, 42, 87, 90, 114, 182, 196, 218, 222, 224, 232, 236
conflict, 10
conscious/consciousness, 3, 10, 12, 14, 30–32, 34–35, 37, 44, 51, 93, 99, 109, 117, 142, 199, 201
clairvoyant consciousness, 104, 112, 129, 219, 223
day consciousness, 108
conscious sin, 192
consciousness soul, 153, 181–182, 194–195
Jesus' replicated consciousness soul, 182
consolidation, 108
Copernicus, 184
corruption, 126
cosmic/cosmos, xiii, 50, 109–110, 116, 119–121, 123, 148–157, 234
rhythm of cosmos, 150–153
courage/courageous, 5–7, 57, 59
creating in the spirit, 232
creation, 46, 94
creation out of nothing, 228, 232–236
Cross (of Christ), 179
crowning with thorns, 52
crying, 205–217
crystalizing, 55
cultural epochs
fifth, 133
customs, 10–11, 27

Damascus, 179

damnation, 215
Darwin, 184
death, 29, 33, 133, 192, 194–195,
    201, 222–223, 437
debility, 78
decay, process, 16
deception, 134
deed, 10
demonic entities, 23
densification, 108
destiny, xviii, 136–137, 140–142, 169,
    195
desire. *See* passion
destruction, 166
deterioration, 190
devachan, 2, 12–13, 29, 37, 41–42,
    45–46, 51, 69–71, 110, 141, 161,
    208, 223–224
    future evil, 13
developmental potential, 221
devil, 127, 133
devotion, 180
Dionysus, 7
disease, xv, 74, 76–84, 95, 102, 111,
    121, 146–148, 158–159, 165,
    167, 169
disharmony, 208–209
dissolution, 184
divine spiritual beings, 92–93,
    109–111, 120, 128–131, 146,
    149–150, 170, 189
division of sexes, 58–59, 102–104,
    107, 111
Dominican, 184
double. *See* phantom
drives, 29, 110, 160, 190, 193, 221
DuBois-Reymond, 184
dynamism, 66

eardrum, 25
earth's catastrophe. *See* atmospheric
    phenomena (earth)
earth's interior (layers), 125, 138–142
    fire earth, 138–139
    forces, 138
Easter, 199
eating, early, 108

Eckhart, Meister, 182, 202
educate/education, 218, 222
egoism/egoistical, 6, 72, 75, 124,
    133–134, 185–186, 197, 214,
    216, 235
    spiritual egotism, 46
egoity, 214
Egypt/Egyptian, 28–29, 32–33, 89,
    94–97, 133, 135, 170
elephant, 54
Elizabeth of Thuringia, 181, 203
emotions, 3–4, 6, 10, 51, 70, 118, 153
enlightenment, 168–169
enthusiasm, 186
envy, 99
equilibrium, 21
error, 97, 130, 192–194, 197–198,
    232
esoteric/esoterically, xiii, 17, 19–20,
    23–24, 27, 29, 37, 40–41, 44, 46,
    52, 54, 59, 63, 75, 82–83, 99,
    106, 125, 127, 134–135,
    140–143, 174, 218
    history, 30, 34
    schools, 202
esotericism
    eastern (oriental), 202–203
    western, 202–203
ether, universal, 159
etheric, 8, 48–50, 53–56, 58, 63–64,
    180, 185–187, 219, 225
    envelope, 219
    forces, 50, 52–53
etheric body, 16–17, 43, 48–51,
    53–56, 58–59, 63–71, 76–77,
    81–84, 91–95, 111–114, 116,
    118–122, 124, 134–135,
    144–149, 151, 153–155,
    158–160, 164, 167, 175–180,
    185–187, 190, 193–194, 198,
    210, 213, 219–220, 222–223,
    229
    archetypal, 175–176
    free aspect, 66–68
    Jesus' replicated, 177–180, 182–183
    rhythmic changes, 118, 121–122
    transformed, 187

twenty-eight day cycle, 145
ethical/ethics, xv–xvi, 69, 72, 105, 195,
    200
evolution (unfold), 223–236
evil, 12–13, 130, 162, 190, 192, 194,
    198, 204, 232
    only prevails for a certain period,
    204
eyes, 2, 68

facial expression, 210
faith, 2
faithfulness, 2
Faust/Faustian (Goethe's person),
    125–126, 142
fear, 200
feel/feelings, 3–4, 6–7, 11, 31, 39–41,
    46, 51–53, 60, 67, 70, 95, 100,
    110, 118, 124, 153, 170, 181,
    208, 215–216, 225, 230
    feelings of inwardness, 236
feelers, astral, 9–10, 17
female, early evolution, 58–59, 103,
    107
fertility, 138
fertilization, 22, 59, 104, 108–110,
    220
    powers, 104, 108
fever, 121–122, 145–148, 150
fire, 132, 139
    forces, 132
    mineral, 139
    primeval, 139
fish, 24–26
    air bladder, 25
    gills, 25
    hearing, 25
    longitudinal lines, 24–26
flour, 183
flowers, 16–18, 63, 222
forces, 18–19, 21, 25, 50–52, 55, 116,
    127, 132, 138–139, 146, 149,
    166, 210, 236
    astral, 23, 210
    defensive, 121
    etheric, 50, 52–53
    fire, 132

fire earth, 138
    healing, 114
    negative, 121
    plant, 18
    soul, 165
forgetfulness, 195
forgetting, 63, 67–72
    forgotten image, 67
fortitude, 5–6
fourfold human nature, 76, 78, 85
Francis of Assisi, 181, 203
Franciscan order, 181
free/freedom, 119, 121–122, 128, 130,
    152, 156, 190, 198–199
free being, 93
free deed, 233
fruitfulness, 11–12, 36, 38
fruition/fruits, 70, 167–168, 173, 200

gall bladder, 82–83
Genesis, book of, 87–88
Germanic, 180
giving, 8
glandular system, 158
God, 90–95, 97, 126, 193, 212, 214
    God of Abraham, Isaac and Jacob,
    91
    Godhead, 93
    godliness, 205
    I-God, 94
    image of, 190
    as Jehovah, 97
    Lord God, 212
    temple of God, 111
    Yahweh, 90, 94, 97
    Yahweh-God, 90–91, 95–97, 99,
    128
Goethe, 11, 16, 103, 125–126,
    133–134, 227
    fairy tale, 39
    Faust, 52, 77, 125–127, 134
    enemy of light, 126
    sons of God of Light, 126
    as Faust poet, 133
    'Prologue in Heaven', 126
    'Realm of the Mothers', 126
Golgotha, event of, 34, 37–38, 101,

133, 180, 196–197, 199–200,
203
goodness, 232
goodwill, 140
Graeco-Roman, 32–37, 133, 135, 170,
231
Greece/Greek, 32, 34–35, 133, 170
grief, 209, 215
group soul (animals), 205, 208–209,
212
group souls (human), 55–60
bull, 56–60
eagle, 56–58
lion, 56–60
man, 56–57
growth, 65–66
grudges, harbouring, 69

habits, 64–65, 167
Haeckel, 184
Ham (son of Noah), 174
harmonize/harmony, 11, 14–15, 24,
111, 120, 122, 126, 146, 151,
153, 156, 167–168, 232
harmony of the spheres. See music of the
spheres
head (human), 54–55, 78, 194, 219
headache, xvi, 52
Hebrew, 87, 97, 126, 133, 174,
176–177
healing, xv, 53, 69, 84, 114, 121, 166
dietic, 84
healing fluidae, 95
hearing, 25, 48
heart organization, 57, 78, 80–82, 112
Heliand Poem, 179–180
hereditary/heredity, 64, 79, 82,
164–165, 167
hermaphrodite, 103–104
bisexual, 59
Hermes, 33, 36, 196
rites of, 170
hierarchical/higher beings. See divine
spiritual beings
hindrances, 141–142, 162
history, 27–29, 33, 52, 183–184
holistic, 84

holy spirit, 199–200, 203, 232–233
leader of 'lodge of twelve', 200
as resurrected luciferic spirit, 199
tongues of fire, 200
Homer, 216
hope, 236
Hussites, 183
Huxley, 184
hydrocephalus, 55
as water on the brain, 55
hydrogen, 48
Hyperborean epoch, 150

I (ego), xvii, 5–7, 23, 30–31, 54–57, 60,
76–80, 83–84, 89–99, 116–118,
120–121, 144–145, 148,
154–155, 158–160, 175–177,
179–182, 185–187, 190,
194–195, 197–198, 208–217,
219, 221–222, 228–230
day I, 117
ego-hood, 214–215
group I, 124, 208–209, 212
I aura, 112
I-bearer, 79, 90
I configuration, 116, 187
I-consciousness, 31
I entity, 208
I-hood, 208
I impulse, 95–96, 98, 100–101
I nature, 216
I point, 95
I power, 98–100
I-realization, 91
as individual, 55
night I, 117
one-day cycle, 145
restricted I, 117
rhythm, 120–121, 123
seat in consciousness soul, 182
true I, 97, 219
universal (great) I, 117
ideas, 3, 5, 7, 9, 30, 62–63, 65–67, 69,
72, 90, 160, 164
ideals, 6, 51
illness, xv–xvii, 7, 66, 71, 73–76,
83–84, 87, 91–92, 95, 102, 109,

111, 121, 159, 161, 165–166, 168–170, 191, 194,
  children, 167
illusion, 32, 134–135, 137, 142, 192, 194, 198, 200
images, 3, 41–42, 65, 68, 71, 94–95, 109, 111
imagination/imaginative, 41, 211, 215
  pictorial/pictures, 44, 51
Imagination (stage), 41, 45–46
imaginative perception, 41, 215
imitative, 106
immersion, 117–118
immorality, 202
impenetrability, 8, 11, 18
impression, 62–63, 65–69
impulses, 51
incorporate/incorporation, 13, 120, 182, 185, 233
India (ancient)/Indian, 29, 31, 33, 131, 133, 135, 196, 231
individuality/individualization, 30, 46, 51, 90, 106–108, 110–111, 156, 167, 176–177, 206–207, 235
infold. *See* involution
inheritance, 206–207
  inherited property, 98
initiate/initiation, 33–34, 36, 44–45, 129, 136, 141–142, 168
  Atlantean, 129, 131
  black magic, 131, 135
  Christian, 52
inner tolerance, 60
Inspiration (stage), 41–43, 45–46
inspire/inspiration, 203, 232
instincts, 10, 64, 109, 128–129, 160, 173–175, 185, 221
Intuition (stage), 41
involution (infold), 223–224, 228, 233–234, 236
Irenaeus, 178

Japheth (son of Noah), 174
Jehovah. *See* God, as Jehovah
jellyfish, 22
Jesus (of Nazareth), 37, 174, 177–180–184, 203

Jewish people, 90–96, 98–100
  as people of Israel, 93
Job, 126
Job, book of, 126
John, St, the Divine, 203
joy, 3, 17–18, 34, 53, 71, 83, 162, 212, 216
Judaism, 180
judgement, power of, 83–184, 226
Jupiter (sphere), 82
Jupiter epoch, 45, 155, 227
justice
  being of, 5, 8
  concept of, 5, 8

kamaloca, 13, 29, 37, 43–45, 49, 51, 69–71, 160–164
karma/karmically, xv–xvi, 84, 136–137, 139–142, 158, 159–169, 192–194, 196–198, 203, 225–226, 229–234
  future karma, 137
Kant-Laplace theory, 149
kidneys, 82
killing (murder), 89, 98–99
knowledge, 27, 53, 62, 115, 183–184, 188, 202
  prophetic, 57

Last Supper, 183
laughing and weeping, 205–208, 211–217
laughter, 205, 207–217, 229
  bleating laughter, 213
  feeling superior, 214
Law of Hammurabi, 100
lawfulness, 229–230, 232
  inner, 47, 65
leaf/leaves, 16–18, 63–64, 222
Lemuria/Lemurian (epoch), 55–56, 102–103, 107, 127–128, 130–131, 139, 150, 170, 172, 189–191, 193–194
Lethe's flood, 70
lies, 194, 198
Life Spirit (Buddhi), 93, 154–155, 186
light, 37, 43, 223, 235

world of, 129
lily of the valley, 222–223, 225, 233
line of descent. *See* hereditary/heredity
lion, 56–60
   lion hearted, 58
   lion race/type, 58–60
liver, 77, 82
locomotor ataxia, 82
logic, 229
Louis the Pious, 179
love, 7, 32, 99
   passionate, 109
   Platonic, 109
   supersensible, 109
Lucifer/luciferic, 127–131, 134, 194,
   196, 198
   bearer of light (light-bearer), 199
   luciferic beings, 189–191, 193,
   198–199
   precedes Christ with flaming torch,
   199
   resurrected, 199
   will have holy spirit, 199
lungs, 82, 121–122, 146

madness. *See* mental illness
magnetism (in earth), 138
male, early evolution, 58–59, 103, 107
manas. *See* Spirit Self (manas)
marriage, 99
Mars (sphere), 82–83
Masters of Wisdom and of the
   Harmony of Feelings, 45–46,
   199–200, 235
materialism/materialistic, xvi, 10,
   75–77, 80–81, 84–85, 95, 126,
   133, 142, 145, 149, 185, 188,
   195, 200
materiality, 104–105, 192
maya. *See* illusion
medicine, 66, 84–85, 124, 201
   herbal, 114
   materialistic, 114
   medical papacy, 75
   mineral-based, 112–113
   creates a phantom-like figure,
   112–114

Melchizedek, 176–177
memory, 62–71, 167, 178-179
mental illness, 6, 23, 123, 165
mental pictures, 4, 7, 44, 67, 95
Mephistopheles/Mephistophelean,
   125–127, 133–135, 189, 194
   spirits of Satan (ahrimanic), 192
Mercury (sphere), 82
messengers of the gods, 35–36
   as an initiate, 36
metabolism, 50
metamorphosis. *See* transform/
   transformation
mid-brain, 166
Middle Ages, 181
mind soul (intellectual/rational), 153,
   181–182, 194, 198
mineral kingdom, 81, 83, 94,
   112–114, 130, 137
Minorites, 181
mobile/mobility, 68, 210, 213
moon (sphere), 13, 82, 107, 120,
   149–151
   separation, 127
Moon, old (ancient), 13, 92, 120, 146,
   148, 152, 155, 185, 190, 193,
   226–229, 232
moral/morality, xvi–xvii, 69, 72, 230
morphology, 124
Moses, 33, 87, 90–91, 94, 96–99, 101,
   196
   Law of Moses, 100
   Mosaic, 100
   pre-Mosaic, 90
movement, organs of, 20–23, 57
murder. *See* killing
music, spiritual, 41–42
music of the spheres, 41, 46
Mystery of Golgotha, 34, 37, 101

nature, 81, 103, 130, 132, 137, 141,
   153–154, 175
nephesh, 212, 214
nerves, 80
nervous/vascular system, 78, 80, 116,
   147, 158
Nietzsche, Friedrich, 6

nitrogen, 48
Noah, 174
nourishment/nutrition, 21–23, 57,
    104, 235
    nutritional juices, 104, 108
    organ of nutrition, 21

obedience, 111
object, 10, 40, 68
    objective/objectively, 40, 45
    objectivizing, 53
obscurity, 197
observations, 19, 25, 29, 40, 48, 78,
    87–88, 103, 114, 123, 158, 206,
    229
obstacles, 162–163
Old Testament, 91, 101, 212
opinion, 10–11
original sin, 110–111, 114
Ormuzd, 32
Osisis, 196
oxygen, 48

pain, 48–50, 52–53, 191–192,
    194–195, 212, 216
    path of knowledge, 52
    suppressed activity, 50
Palestine, 178–180
Pancreas, 77
Papias, 178
Paracelsus/Paracelsian, 85
paroxysm, 148
passions, 29, 64, 70, 109–112,
    128–129, 138–139, 160, 190,
    193, 195, 198, 221
pathology, 124
patience, 15
Paul, St/Pauline, 179
    as Saul, 179
penetrability, 8
perceive/perception, 4, 17, 21, 24,
    30–31, 33, 41, 49, 52–53, 90,
    118, 128, 130–131, 133, 141,
    156, 198–199, 201–202, 215,
    227
    clairvoyant, 104, 180
    imaginative, 41

spiritual, 84
permeability, 8
Persia (ancient)/Persian, 28–29, 32,
    131–133, 135, 196, 231
personality, 2, 31, 34, 40, 181
    endowed with, 136
Peter, St, 178
phantom (demon), 134–135, 137
phantom (double), 112–114, 135
phenacetin, 124
philosophic/philosophy, 6, 78, 103,
    201
physical body, as temple of God, 111
physiology, 77
pictorial image. *See* mental picture
picture. *See* mental picture
plant kingdom, 16–20, 30, 63–65,
    67–68, 81, 83, 94, 130, 132, 192,
    220, 222, 224, 233
    forces, 18
    infolding, 223
    sexual maturation, 220–221
    soul nature, 17–18
    unfolding, 223
pleasure, 225
pneumonia, 115, 121–122, 145
    seventh day is crisis, 115, 122,
        145–146, 154
Polaric epoch, 150
pressure, differences in water, 24–25
primal powers, 152
primum mobile, xvii, 149
privation, 43–44, 46, 49–52, 70–71
Protestant, 234
psyche, 6, 83
psychic, 6, 76, 58
psychological/psychology, 48, 83–84,
    113
puberty, 105, 219–220

Raphael, 227
rapture, 23
realm of shades, 35, 38, 133, 197
reason, 206
recapitulation, 63–64
reciprocal, 76, 82, 104, 107, 109–110
redeem/redemption, 87, 199

reincarnate/reincarnation, 133, 160, 166, 172, 176
religion, 75
renunciation, 44–46, 52
repetition, 16–17
replicate/replication (multiplies), 63, 121, 175–177, 182
reproduce/reproduction, 20, 22–23, 57, 59–60, 63, 104
resemblance, 52
retrogression, 193
revenge, 5
reverberation, 20
reverent, 60
rhythm (cycle)/rhythmically, 118–120, 122–124, 144–156
    animal bodies, 124
    birth/conception rhythm, earlier, 152
    human bodies, 118–123, 144–145
riddles, unresolved, 62
rigidity, 210
Rishis, Holy, 33–34, 196
Roman, 32
roots, 63, 222
rose, 17, 41, 67–68
ruin, 132

sacrifice, 46, 235
    self-sacrifice, 46
salt, 55
    crystallizing, 55
Saturn (sphere), 82
Saturn, old (ancient), 46, 81, 92, 120, 138, 148, 152, 155, 185, 189, 193, 226–229, 231–233
Savonarola, 51
Scholaticism, 181–182, 184
Schopenhauer, 105
scourge, 50
seed, 37, 64–65, 71, 220, 222–223
    potencies, 132
self-awareness, 6, 57, 31, 54, 97–98.
    See also I (ego)
self-creation, 233
semblance, 52
sensory/sensory world, xv, 2, 14–15,

31, 34–35, 40, 76, 97, 108–110, 128, 130–131, 134, 137, 145, 172, 191–192, 195, 198, 200, 227, 231
sentient/sentience, 3, 188
sentient soul, 153, 181, 194
    Jesus' sentient soul, 181
sentiment, 4
sexual drive, 109–110
Shankaracharya, 203
Shem (Noah's son)/Semitic, 174–177
Shiva (Indian religion), 166
sickness. *See* illness
sight, 48
sin, 192, 194, 198–199
    original sin, 87
Siphonophora, 21, 23
sleep, 3, 30–31, 116–118, 123, 129, 144, 150, 159
    sleep consciousness, 31
smell, 48
smiling, 215–216
somnambulistic, 134
sound, 41
soul, 3–5, 7–8, 11, 15, 17–18, 28–30, 36–37, 39, 45–46, 60, 64–67, 72, 83, 89, 91, 95–96, 99, 113–115, 124, 128–129, 133, 138, 142, 155–156, 161, 163–166, 168–169, 173, 187–189, 194, 197, 200–202, 210, 212, 214, 225, 227
    soul, possessions, 227
    soul-spiritual, 173
speed of rotation, 145
spirit/spiritual, xvii, 1–3, 7, 11–12, 14–15, 17, 23, 25, 28–39, 41, 45–46, 52, 55–56, 58–61, 64, 66–67, 69, 72, 75–76, 79–81, 83, 85, 88, 93, 96, 98–100, 103, 105, 108–111, 114, 116, 120, 124–131, 133–135, 137–138, 152, 154–157, 159–161, 164–165, 173, 177, 185–186, 189, 191–192, 195–198, 200–202, 205, 208–209, 214–215, 223–224, 232, 235

spirit as *primum mobile*, 121
spiritual perception, 84
spiritual substantiality, 51
Spirit Man (Atma), 155, 186–187
Spirit Self (Manas), 93, 154–155, 186
Spirits of Form, 189–191
spirits of light, 136
Spirits of Movement, 189–190
Spirits of Personality, 189, 228–231,
    234–235
  as powers of personality, 228
  as Spirits of Time, 231
  as Time Spirits, 231
spirits of Satan, 189
Spirits of Wisdom, 46, 189–190
spiritual economy, 176
spiritual science. *See* anthroposophical/
    anthroposophy
spleen, 82
Steiner, Marie, xiii
Steiner, Rudolf
  'The Bible and Wisdom', 87
  Cosmic Memory, 132
  The Education of a Child, 194
  'Interior of the World', 141
  Knowledge of the Higher Worlds, xiii
  The Stages of Higher Knowledge, xiii
  Theosophy, xiii, 193, 201
  'Where and How Do We Find the
    Spirit', xiii
stems, 222
stomach, 78, 80
Strauss, David Friedrich, 184
submersion, 117–118
substantiality, 18–19, 21–22
suffering, xv, 17–18, 50, 52, 70–71,
    191–192, 194–195
sun (sphere), 13, 82, 108, 120, 122,
    131, 138, 151, 185
  separation, 131, 136, 148
  spiritual sun, 108
  when it didn't turn on its axis,
    120–121
Sun, old (ancient), 46, 92, 148, 152,
    155, 185, 190, 193, 226–229,
    232–233
sun spirits, 120

sunrise, effect of, 107
supersensible, 27, 95, 97, 109, 149,
    174, 177, 200
superstition, 115
sympathetic/sympathy, 32, 34–36, 40,
    216

Tabes, 82
tableau (memory panorama), 29, 36,
    69, 159, 167
taste, 43
  taste experience, 20
Tauler, Johannes, 182
temperaments, 65, 71–72, 206
  melancholic, 71–72, 165
  phlegmatic, 71–72
  sanguine, 71–72
Ten Commandments, 74, 84, 87–92,
    94, 96–97, 100–102
  German version, 88
  as progenitor of Semitic race,
    174–176
Theosophical Society, xiii
  Besant branch, xiii
  German section, xiii, 73
theosophy, xiii
therapy, 124
thinking, 8, 11–12, 15, 40–42, 76, 85,
    141, 153–154, 164, 182, 184,
    187, 229–231, 235
  lawful (logical), 229–230, 232
  materialistic, 133, 149
  objective, 41
thinking, feeling, will, 39, 156
thoughts, 3–4, 8–10, 40–41, 51, 62,
    75, 99, 102, 152, 154–155, 157,
    176, 184–185, 229, 234–235
tolerance, 11
tone, 41–42
  spiritual, 46
torment, 70
transform/transformation, 16–17,
    21–22, 40–41, 44–46, 51, 58,
    60, 67, 71, 77, 154–155, 179,
    187, 195, 199, 208, 222
transgressions, 95
transition, 53, 69, 91, 181–182

Thrones (spirits), 46, 189, 228–229
truth, 11, 35, 37, 41, 172, 180,
    182–183, 202–203, 232
twins, 20

unconscious/unconsciousness, 117, 145
unfold. *See* evolution (unfold)
unity, 6, 23, 31, 56

vanity, 142–143
Venus (sphere), 82
Venus epoch, 45, 155, 227–228
vertebrae, 63
virtues, 234
Vishvakarman, 196
visions, 51, 58
Vulcan epoch, 155, 227, 233, 235

warmth, 49
weeping. *See* crying
Whitsun, 199
will, 39–41, 46, 184, 188, 200–201
    impulse, 3
    will to learn, 184

wisdom, 84, 103, 155–156, 184–185,
    198–200
    esoteric, 203
    wisdom-imbued, 199
withered, 69
Word. *See* Christ, Word
world-view, 15–16, 34, 76, 88, 153,
    188, 195, 202
    anthroposophic, 62, 188, 202, 218
    idealism, 188
    materialism, 188
    monism, 188
    realism, 188
    spiritualism, 188
worry, 68

Yahweh, 90, 94, 97
Yahweh-God, 90–91, 95–97, 99

Zarathustra, 33, 36, 131–132
zeitgeist, 231
Zoroastrian culture, 133
Zwingli, 183